YOUR
TOXIC ENEMY

UNLOCK THE KEY TO GETTING YOUR HEALTH RIGHT!

JUDIE DIETZLER

To order additional copies of this book, contact:
Bookwhip
1-855-339-3589
https://www.bookwhip.com

CONTENTS

To everyone who has had a chronic diagnosed or misdiagnosed illnesses:

You have had an inner voice that has said you are tired, sick, or not feeling well, and you feel there is a physical problem, and you go to your doctor and list your complaints and symptoms hoping he or she will diagnose the problem and help you find the solution so you will once again be "Healthy." But so many times what happens is that instead of getting a diagnosis, finding a solution and regaining your health, you walk out of the doctor's office with prescriptions for the symptoms that you listed, which in many cases will add to your health problems over time.

I am giving a voice to the millions of people who have walked into a doctor's office, desperate for help, only to walk out with a handful of prescriptions that will give them more reasons to visit a doctor in desperation. What they need is someone who will take the time to help them find the answers to the questions they've had for a very long time.

This book will help you on your journey toward recovery and renewed health.

FOREWORD

This book is a testament to two important journeys of discovery that merged together over a period of twenty- three years for Judie Dietzler. The first was as a very healthy woman who suddenly developed an unknown, stabbing pain in both thumb joints so severe that she couldn't use her hands without wearing special braces. If that were the only problem, she would have ignored it like so many people do, and blamed it on genetics or lifestyle, but less than a year later, she developed a neurological problem so severe that there was no way she could ignore it.

She did what most people do when they get sick. She went to the doctor. The doctors did what they were trained to do. They ran tests and examined her, but all of the tests came back normal. Because they could not link any of their medical tests or exams to an illness, they assumed Mrs. Dietzler was depressed, so they wanted to prescribe antidepressants.

Mrs. Dietzler is well qualified on the topic of toxic chemicals as someone who has lived with neurotoxicity for over two decades, who can share first hand knowledge and experiences of the devastation and havoc that just a little amount of toxins can cause when exposed to the human body.

She can also speak as a clinical hypnotherapist who has worked with many patients over the years who have been exposed to toxic chemicals with equally devastating results. Several friends and clients will share their heartwarming stories about how they dealt with chemical exposure.

And for the past two decades, she has also researched toxic chemicals, which led her to discover the true source of her toxic exposure and the way to remove the toxins from her body.

Mrs. Dietzler was a sales director with a top cosmetic firm for over twenty years, which gave her a strong work ethic, motivation, and a very positive attitude that would carry her through adversity. As a hypnotherapist, she is trained to teach people how to listen to the body as their guide.

Both careers, along with her years as a medical technologist, gave her the innate ability to always research subjects completely. For the past twenty years, she spent countless hours researching until she was finally able to put all of the pieces together so she could begin the healing process.

She has been symptom-free for over eight years, but through her research for the book, she discovered she was not alone in her journey. Many people are walking the same toxic path that she did, feeling alone without anyone to talk to about their problems. Their doctors give them medication, exacerbating the problem. Their friends start to think they are hypochondriacs, and spouses are tired of listening to their complaints. They even begin to doubt themselves. Don't question your sanity. Read Judie's story and see if you can find a piece of you inside.

This book is timely. Judie spent twenty years hiding her story from everyone, but through her research and the loss of a close friend, she decided she needed to share her narrative. She hopes that, by sharing her story, she may be able to help you find the solution to your health problem. She shows you how you can take easy steps to go from harm to healing.

God bless you on your journey.

PREFACE

I have found that things are not always as they seem. You have to be willing to step out of your comfort zone and ask questions and keep asking until you find the right answers. At times in emergency situations, you need a doctor to make a split-second decision and prescribe a medication, but that is not always the case when you have a long-term chronic mystery illness.

Each of us is taken down the path we are on for a reason, and it is not for me to question the reason I am on this route. What is important is that I learn from the journey and I share what I've learned with others.

When illness strikes, it demands that we make a choice. We can choose to listen only to our traditionally trained medical doctor and follow his or her instructions explicitly, or we can listen to our own inner wisdom. I wrote this book for those who are sick with an undiagnosed illness and still don't know why but are determined to find the answer and solution.

As a hypnotherapist, I believe that all problems have a solution, but you need to be willing to put forth the effort required to find the answer. There is not one person who has more of a vested interest in your health than you do, so you should be willing to do the legwork. It will require more than picking up the phone and calling your traditional medical doctor, going in for your fifteen- minute token visit, and getting your new prescription that will make your problem worse.

Life is a series of causes and effects, and your health is the same. You are presently dealing with the effect of the problem so you need to go back in time and determine the initial cause (when it started). Once you decide that, you can begin the healing process. Together we will begin the step- by-step process showing you how to determine what caused your illness. I will show you the way, but you will need to do the work.

You will go on my journey through harm's way. I will share stories of a few friends and clients, but I won't leave you hanging. I will share how I found my way to healing after two decades. I won't sugarcoat it. It wasn't easy. Nothing worthwhile is usually easy, but it paid dividends.

The information inside this book could hold the key to your mystery undiagnosed illness. Inside your body, you may have an uninvited house guest, neurotoxin (a substance that is poisonous or destructive to nerve tissue), endocrine disruptors (a cause for cancerous tumors, birth defects, and other developmental disorders), or carcinogens (substances capable of causing cancer). If the tests say you're normal, the doctor thinks you're depressed, and you feel like your body is falling apart, this book is for you.

Here are just a few possible symptoms from toxic chemical exposure:

sleep disorder
pain
cancer
attention deficit disorder (ADD) or attention deficit/ hyperactivity disorder (ADHD)
Parkinson's or Alzheimer's disease multiple sclerosis (MS) amyotrophic lateral sclerosis (ALS)
fatigue
infertility
unexplained weight gain fibromyalgia
allergies
blurred vision
angina
cataracts

colitis

constipation

depression

eye or lung damage headaches/migraines indigestion/acid reflux

lack of concentration

loss of hair, memory, or libido nerve or neurological disorders protein/
sugar in urine

seizures

skin ailments/rashes

tumors

This only gives you a random sample of how a little amount of toxins over time can affect the human body.

Your Toxic Enemy will help guide you step-by-step and show you that healing is possible, but it will ultimately be your responsibility to do the required work to begin the healing process. I have helped many people walk the path to healing, including myself, and I know you can do it.

ACKNOWLEDGMENTS

Until almost eight years ago, my life, as far as my health was concerned, was in limbo. I knew I had a problem, and six months earlier, it had once again escalated to the point where I was leaving several of my beloved organizations because of my neurotoxicity. In twenty years, it was a secret I only shared with two people, and I trusted them with my life. When I was sick, I would vanish and reappear when I was feeling normal. (My husband may dispute the normal part.)

Almost eight years ago my son, Tyson Schmidt, reintroduced me to a chemical- free product called Melaleuca. I had heard of Melaleuca when I first started having symptoms, but I didn't realize neurotoxicity caused my problems, so I didn't think I would ever find a solution. Fast-forward twenty years after two decades of research, tons of money spent on doctors, medicine, tests, and blood work with no results, and I am motivated.

The information I received about the products impressed me. The company was a manufacturing company, but unlike others like them, they only manufactured toxic-free products. I started using the products and removed all of the toxic products in my home, and little by little, my symptoms lessened. She has been symptom-free since 2011.

I would like to thank so many people that helped me start on my journey to healing. Dr. Mike McCullough, Margie Rae, Mitch Tippetts, and Susie Rohnert, you shared your wealth of knowledge about household chemicals and gave me the curiosity to put together the final pieces of the puzzle to start my healing process. If my son, Tyson, had not invited me over to his house for a Barbecue I wound't have met Mitch and got started on the road to healing. For that, I will be eternally grateful. I would also like to thank Capstone Services for their help, along with all the previous people who have cared enough to research about toxic chemicals, write articles and books, and spread the word.

I would also like to thank all of the companies that develop chemical-free products. If consumers refuse to buy products that are harming their families, manufacturers will listen because it affects their bottom line. They produce the products we buy, and we are in the driver's seat. My husband and I, my son and grandchildren have chemical-free homes.

Because I have neurotoxicity, one of the symptoms is memory confusion and a disconnect in the brain, so it was important for me to find one company that had chemical- free household, body and hair care, and cosmetic products. I only wanted to work with one company.

Many companies make chemical-free products. It's not important where you get your products. What is important is that you use chemical-free products.

INTRODUCTION

As you read through the chapters, you will find my story and the narrative of others who have had similar challenges and struggles that you have gone through, but as you continue to read, I believe you will also find pieces of you scattered throughout the chapters because much of our tears and pain are the same.

If you haven't already started keeping a journal, now would be a good time to start because my words will help spark your own wonderful ideas that hold the key to unlock the solution to your healing.

Most of my life, I have been led to believe that my doctor could solve my problems. Thinking was never part of the equation. I just picked up the phone when I didn't feel well and went to see the doctor. As soon as I walked into his office, I immediately went into hypnosis. I didn't ask one question, hung on every word he said, and walked out with a toxic prescription.

Years later after I became a hypnotist, someone would say, "I can't be hypnotized."

I would say, "You've gotta be kidding. That's the craziest thing I've ever heard. Why don't I just go to the doctor with you the next time and we will test that theory?"

Your doctor will not solve your health problems. His job is usually to keep you at status quo, which is not healthy. The best I can determine is that it is somewhere between fogging a mirror and neutral. The best you will ever get as to the "How is my health, doc?" response is "Normal," but he will usually follow it with "for a woman your age." You're not sure if you should cry or kiss him, but there's no need to worry about doing either one. Your fifteen minutes is over, and you are shuffled out of the office.

So if your goal is health, you are on the right track. You've bought this book. You have either a pen and paper or a journal in hand to take notes, and hopefully, your mind is clear of clutter. So as I go through my journey in *Your Toxic Enemy*, you will start remembering your past and the toxins that might have crept into your life.

As I begin working on solutions to heal from all of the toxins in my environment, you will also inventory your life, friendships, relationships, environment, and home and determine which toxins you need to eliminate. Next, you will evaluate what you need to do to remove the toxic chemicals that are currently in your body and which lifestyle changes you may need or want to make in order to ultimately be healthy. After you've finished the evaluations and made the appropriate adjustments, how will you feel? Proud. You've accomplished so much more than if you had just sat in the doctor's office waiting for a toxic prescription.

Will you never go to a doctor? No. I am going to show you how to find a doctor who will take the time to find the cause of your health problems and determine a solution. You need a doctor who understands toxic chemicals and knows how to test for them and treat a patient who has toxicity.

Will the work be worth it? A resounding yes. Will you make any sacrifices as you go through the steps to regain your health? Depends on how you look at it. I had to let a good friend go. She was just too toxic for me.

It's your health and your life. You have a vested interest in the outcome.

1

LIFE HAPPENS WHEN YOU HAVE OTHER PLANS

I decided to write this book out of necessity because I've had a long, difficult, twenty-three-year journey that I never planned to take, but life sometimes happens as you are making other plans.

My first thought is that the pain is too great for too long. It's time to end the fight. I've lost my best friend. Only two people know what I've been going through for the past several years. I keep a happy face for the world, but I'm falling apart inside. Darrel was the best friend I ever had. He died suddenly in 2003, but I never completely recovered from the loss of having such a wonderful friend. When you are sick for so long, it makes your thinking fuzzy, your emotions are all over the place, and you are just a little abnormal.

If you're feeling abnormal, this book is right up your alley. So why is this book important? I finally decided to break my silence and tell my story for two reasons:

- I spent twenty years going to traditional doctors and spending countless hours, wasted time, and thousands of dollars out of my own pocket to be told that all of the tests were normal. They couldn't find anything wrong, but they had many options for the pain, nausea, insomnia, indigestion, and so forth. In the meantime, I kept getting worse until I felt that my nameless illness was hopeless. I didn't have anyone I felt I could talk to about my unknown illness, including my doctors. How do you talk to someone who only allows you fifteen minutes for your office visit? And of course, at the end of your visit, you can count on two more prescriptions to keep you company. I finally realized that, if I had been running in circles for twenty years, exposed to toxic chemicals, and unable to get any help, there must be hundreds or thousands of other people with a mystery illness who are equally frustrated that also need help.

- If you are sick and have had a similar experience, you can relate to my story. You have probably been searching for many of the same answers because, as time progresses, toxic chemical symptoms seem to blend together so you may find parts of your life as you turn the pages of my book, which may lead you to your own answers.

I take you on my journey through the pain, the anger, the frustration, the research, the aha moments, and finally the wisdom and healing. You will see into the depths of my despair, but you will also see when I finally walked into the sunshine and realized that, for the first time in many years, there is real hope. Life is great and both you and I have the potential to live a long, healthy life. Let's journey together and travel from harm to healing.

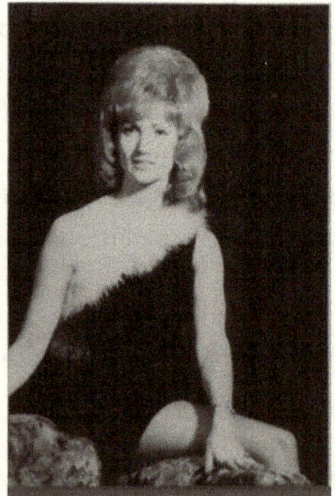

Judie In photo beauty contest in 1975

At the time, I was a senior sales director with a top cosmetics company and traveled extensively with my business. I had been one of the seminar speakers in front of hundreds of women for several years and had won cars, diamonds, and furs.

I began my career in 1975 when Mary Kay Cosmetics was sponsoring a photo beauty contest in Wichita, Kansas, and I was asked to participate. I was so shy and quiet, but I said I would do it.

Mary Kay wasn't an easy career move for me, and sales were an even harder transition. I was like a fish out of water. I didn't have girlfriends and only hung out with guys. I was a medical technologist. I had only been married to my second husband for three months. I was looking for something I could do while my son was in school and I could be at home when he was there, so Mary Kay looked like the ideal career.

Two years earlier, when my son was only three years old, his dad asked to spend the day with him while I was at work, and when I got home, he had vanished with him, along with all of his belongings and his newborn puppies. That was the last I saw of my son until he was almost five years old when the police said we could pick him up in Grand Portage, Minnesota (a hundred miles from Canada). I'd spent almost two years searching in desperation, so now that I had him back, I was afraid to let him out of my sight. I worked when he was in school and took him with me to every Mary Kay function, including sales meetings, and he sat quietly drawing pictures.

I hated talking to strangers, and I wasn't crazy about sales. But I did have two wonderful mentors, Mary Kay Ash and Ila Burgardt, who became my national sales director. I knew I could win if I had them on my side. I was determined to be a success. Staying home with my son was that important to me.

Zig Ziglar once said that salesmen are not born, but they do die, so somewhere along the way, they become salesmen. I listened to the advice of my mentors and became a director in eleven months. In 1976, I moved to Idaho, along with two of my consultants, to build the business as the first director in Idaho. We made a huge splash, and soon we had a pink Cadillac. I never forgot the many inspirational letters I received from Mary Kay over the years, letting me know how proud she was of my achievements.

But the one lesson I learned the hard way because of my illness and my twenty-five years devoted to just a single company is to never put all of your eggs in one basket. Always have more than one source of income so that, if anything happens to your primary paycheck, you will have money from other directions, whether it is from a second business, network marketing, an affiliate business, investments, an annuity, and so forth. I wish someone had given me that advice.

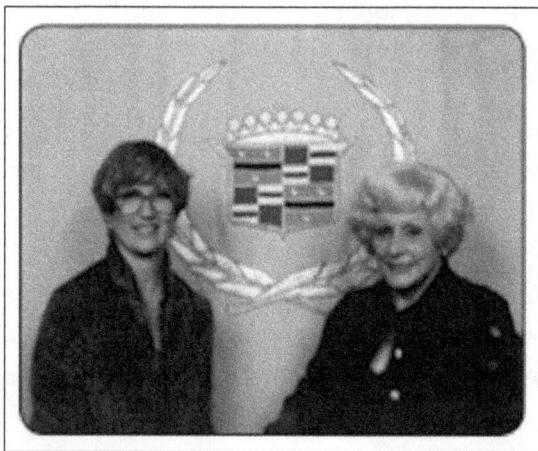

My mentor and initial sales trainer, Mary Kay Ash.

I truly thought my life was good and could only get better.

MY DIRECTOR TRAINING CLASS WITH MARY KAY ASH IN 1976

But unfortunately, life does change, and it doesn't always go the direction you would like. I was doing a presentation onstage in 1990 in front of a group when I suddenly got dizzy, lost my balance, and fell off the stage. From that day on, my life was never the same. I remember how quickly I tried to regain my composure after the incident, thinking it was only a temporary problem. Fortunately, it was the end of

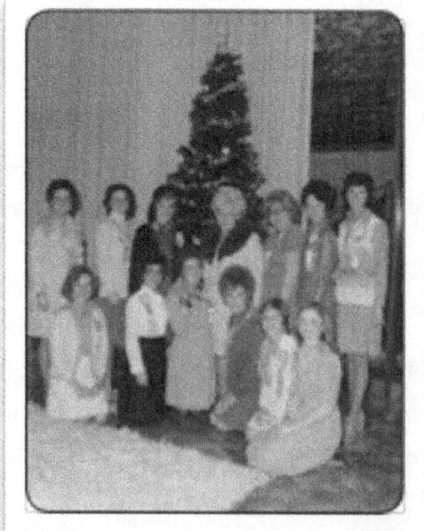

the presentation, so most of the audience was unaware that there was a real problem. I recovered most of my dignity. I was still feeling the effects when I got home, so I rested the rest of the day, and the next day, I was fine without another problem for a couple weeks.

But I kept having the strange balance and brain problems, and I had to either cancel business appointments or reschedule them.

I had symptoms of a stroke several times a month, and I was referred to every type of available specialist. My condition baffled every doctor I had an appointment with, and every consultation became a little more frustrating. I had the opportunity to see almost every neurologist in the area where I live, and each one said a diagnosis would not be a problem if he or she could see me when I was having an episode.

When I had symptoms, my husband would rush me to the office, and we were told that the doctor had absolutely no time to see us, but he or she had an opening in six weeks and would be happy to schedule me even though the likelihood of my symptoms magically reappearing at the new appointment time was pretty slim.

Each time I saw any doctor, I would give him or her my symptoms and always walk out of his or her office with a prescription for each symptom unless I refused to take it, which was often the case with me.

I would first say, "I am having problems sleeping." The doctor would ask, "Are you depressed?" I would say, "No."

The doctors gave me a prescription for Ambien for sleep and an antidepressant. So the roller coaster began. I was not getting better but much worse. On some days, I would literally crawl my way to the bathroom.

Four months into my illness, I received a call from the vice president of the company that I had devoted twenty-five years of my life to and had planned my retirement around, asking me to resign my position as a senior sales director.

Because I was currently unable to handle the duties I had been doing in the past and it would be unclear if and when I might be able to return, they felt it was best if I resigned from my position. I was self-employed and an independent contractor, and until they said they wanted me to resign, it never crossed my mind that my career was in jeopardy.

I knew that one of the requirements as a director was that I needed to maintain my unit monthly production, and if I didn't sustain it for three months in a row, they could ask me to resign. But I was in a medical crisis and had been with the company for a long time, so I thought they would take that into consideration. But unfortunately, that didn't happen. I had worked since I was sixteen years old, and I'd never had a problem finding a job or launching a career.

I had worked very hard over the years and had many great customers, and even if I were no longer a senior sales director, I could still service my customers, and my husband could help me deliver products to them, so I still had an income. It was much less than I had as a director, but it was a wonderful blessing.

When I was twenty-one years old, I'd enrolled in a Dale Carnegie course that gave me confidence in my abilities early in my life, but Mary Kay had taught me how to set priorities. And right now, rebuilding a new career and income had to be put on the back burner while I put all of my effort into regaining my health. I was sick, not sure what I had, and without a career. My outlook on life felt gloomy, but I knew brighter days were around the corner.

I found that most doctors allowed fifteen minutes to examine and talk to you at your appointment, so I tried to write down my questions so I could get as many answered as possible, but my case was still such a mystery, and the solution was usually to keep giving me medication, which only made the problem worse.

I was tested and probed by family doctors and internists, but mostly by neurologists throughout Idaho, and I even traveled as far as Rush Presbyterian Hospital in Chicago and Mayo Clinic in Phoenix. I was given MRIs to detect structural abnormalities in the body; CT scans to diagnose tumors; fractures, bony structures, and infections in the organs and tissues of the body; PET scans to detect cancer; EEGs of every type to measure and record the electrical activity of my brain; spinal taps to evaluate the fluid surrounding the brain and spinal cord; psychological testing; and blood tests. I had every test imaginable. I was always told that everything was normal except for the EEG, which was always abnormal, but they didn't have an explanation for that.

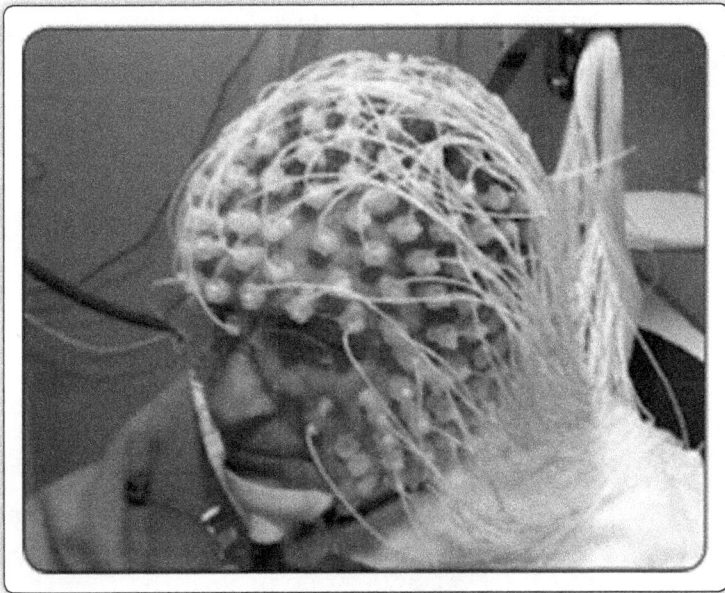

The psychological testing showed a cognitive disconnect between the visual, memory, and concentration with a conclusion of vascular dementia. The MRI I had been told was normal all of these years had a tiny, nonspecific focus of T2 weighted signal abnormality within the left frontal white matter. The radiologist surmised it was likely the result of chronic microvascular disease.

Over the years, at every office visit with many different doctors, I had always taken the reports showing the psychological tests, EEGs, and MRIs all highlighted because I had researched my own case completely. I knew that, out of the thousands of reports and paperwork, the answer was in the information I was presenting to them, but I needed their expertise to help find the answers. But they failed to either care enough or take the time.

Not only did I have neurological problems, I developed pain that traveled throughout my entire body. It started in my thumbs, and it finally got so bad that the hand specialist made special braces out of plaster that I had to wear all of the time to protect my thumbs. I'm still supposed to wear them, but it is impossible to do anything except watch TV and eat bonbons when I wear them, so I cheat most of the time except when I lift heavy stuff like my chunky shih tzus.

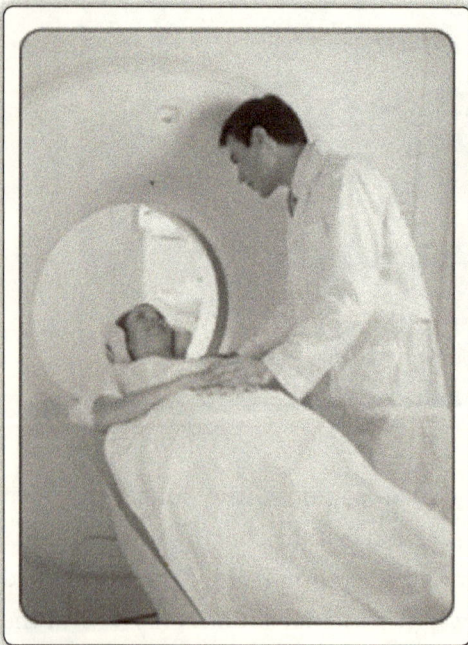

I attended a medical seminar that was being conducted in Boise, and one of the keynote speakers was a doctor from California. He suggested I go to Los Angeles.

The Solution: The Patient Must Become the Student, Teacher, and Healer

I look at life differently than many people. I believe all problems have a solution. It is called cause and effect. In order to solve the problem, you need to first find out what caused the problem. That requires asking questions. When you get the answers to those questions, you need to ask more questions, and you **keep asking questions until you get to the questions that determine when the problem first began.**

The doctors I went to didn't take the time to ask questions. They formed an opinion and diagnosis based on their past experiences, not my experiences. As a result, I continued to get worse because the toxicology panel revealed that I had toxic chemicals in my body, and the medical community was adding an additional toxic overload by prescribing medications that were causing more problems. They were working on the band-aid approach rather than looking at it through the eyes of medical science and thinking that perhaps I had a condition that did not fit into the mold of their normal office visit.

I stayed out of the public eye for close to five years, and when I did take on projects, I always tried to have assignments that gave me the flexibility to leave at the drop of a hat whenever I had a neurological problem. I knew I would need to leave for three or four hours until the problem went away. Only two people were close enough to me to know I had a problem. I lived in silence for over twenty years before I shared my worst fear with anyone besides my husband and a dear friend who died in 2003.

There is a saying, "If it's meant to be, it's up to me," and nothing became truer as I was searching for the answers to regain my health. There were times I had neurological problems daily, and then I would go for a week or two without any symptoms. I kept journals so I could see if I could see a pattern, but there didn't seem to be a set configuration.

I searched the internet to try to find the answers to my nagging questions about toxic chemicals and the way they affect the human body, but I couldn't connect the dots. Through my internet searches, I found many environmental experts that said that if you use chemical-free cleaning, body, and hair care products, it would greatly improve your health, which made sense.

Then something strange happened in June 2011. My son invited me over to his house to a barbecue. While we were there, he told us about a manufacturing company that sold only chemical-free, full-strength concentrated products, and I could order everything I needed from one location, which would save me both time and money. They would ship to my home. They had everything I was looking for, including cleaning, body, hair, and skin products. I decided to give it a try.

As the days and weeks went by, I realized I had not had any neurological problems, but I could sense uneasiness when I went grocery shopping, when the landscaper sprayed chemicals, or when I went into a business that had the smell of chemicals. Slowly, I started to make a connection between my initial chemical exposure in 1990 and the fact that, when I was constantly exposed to toxic chemicals in small doses, it was reinforcing my initial exposure. My body was already in an overload situation and simply could not handle additional exposure, so it was reacting the only way it knew how: shutting down the area that was in toxic overload.

Over the next few months, I started realizing that I had not had any neurological episodes since I had been using toxic-free products from the company that my son recommended to me and I have been symptom free since 2011.

Because I had been using toxic-free products, my head cleared enough that I began researching for the book, which led me to my actual diagnosis and the toxin causing my neurological problems. I also found a way to remove the toxins from my body and regain my health and life permanently. All of that happened because I was led on a journey and I was open enough to pay attention to the signals and listen to the inner voice that helped me along the way.

I have gained some of my confidence back since I haven't had neurological problems for a while. I have given talks in front of groups and been on trips with friends without dragging my husband along as my security blanket, and I feel wonderful.

While doing the research, I discovered that not only were household toxins hurting just my health, they were affecting the health of every other person on the earth. I found that all of the many illnesses that many of us think of as normal may be problems that can and should be avoided.

I would like to share the information so it may help improve your life or the life of someone you love. In 2010, I was in Mayo Clinic for a week, and they finally discovered what I thought was the final element to my condition so we could fill in the blanks of the crossword puzzle. I still had a long way to go before I had a complete understanding of both my illness and the journey to healing.

My original exposure was in 1987. The first symptom was pain in my thumbs, followed by vasculitis. In 1990 I started having Neurological problems.

Within a year after the vasculitis, I had the first neurological symptom. Mayo Clinic diagnosed the problem with the brain as a rare condition that is difficult to diagnose, basilar brainstem migraines. When someone has a basilar migraine, there is a disturbance at the brainstem or base of the brain. Even before the migraine headache begins, the person may experience an aura, a cluster of sensations such as dizziness, double vision, and lack of coordination. An aura is a neurological phenomenon that occurs about ten to forty-five minutes before the headache starts. I finally found a wonderful neurologist who understands basilar migraines, and I have a medication that balances out the migraines. But the key element is reducing my exposure to toxic chemicals.

Chapter 1 Review

1. What is the date of your first symptom? _____

2. List your symptoms: _____
   _____
   _____
   _____

3. List your blood work:
   _____
   _____
   _____

4. List the medications, herbs, products, and so forth you have used.

   Name/date/worked   Name/date/didn't work

   _____.   _____
   _____.   _____
   _____.   _____
   _____.   _____
   _____.   _____

Lessons I've Learned in My Life

Trust is like an eraser; it gets smaller and smaller with every mistake.

2

ENEMY BEHIND CLOSED DOORS!

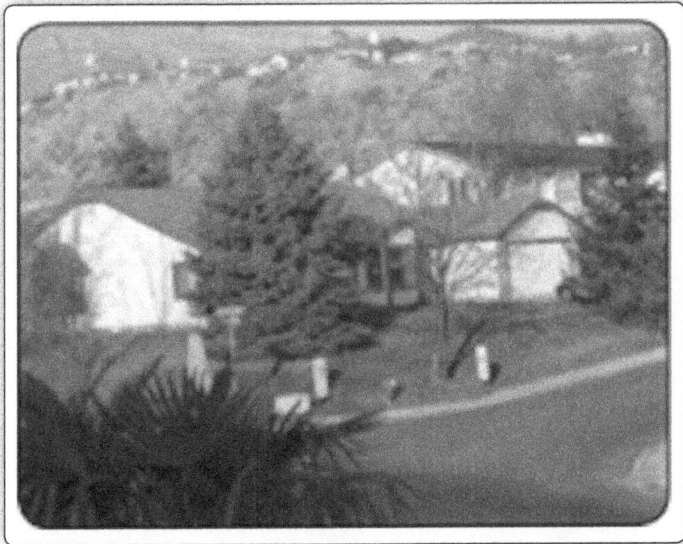

The Home Where I Lived When I First Started Having The Neurological Symptoms

Y ou're always one choice away from changing your life! I remember one night having the opportunity to babysit with my first grandchild, Sky. He was only three months old and such a little sweetheart. I was having a business meeting, and he was lying on the floor on a blanket, taking a nap. He started to wake up, and I leaned down to pick him up when I felt I was having a balance problem. I instantly knew I was having the beginning of neurological problems so I laid him back down and gently rubbed him on his back until he fell back to sleep. I stayed on the floor until the problem went away, and fortunately that night, I wasn't the person in charge of the meeting. After that night, I realized I needed to be careful when I was around my grandchildren and make sure I always had someone who could take over for me.

The following article is an excerpt from the e-book *Healthy Living for a Busy Family*. Dr. George Grant, founder of the International Academy of Wellness, wrote about the dangers in household cleaning products. I would like to dedicate this chapter to excerpts taken from his article.

Are you poisoning your children? Dr. Grant states that it's pretty scary when you think of all those people who use toxic chemicals to clean their homes and don't know the dangers. He used to be one of those people who had no clue that the chemicals he was using were so harmful.

He states that a greater number of children under the age of four die of accidental poisonings at home rather than accidental gunfire at home. The average home today contains more chemicals than are found in a typical chemistry lab. He states that we should go into our kitchen and our bathroom and look under the sinks where we keep our cleaning and personal care supplies. What will we find? Window cleaner? Bleach? Dishwashing detergent? Shampoo? Toothpaste? If we read the label on toothpaste, *it says not to swallow the paste.*

He then states that these products can be violent, lethal poisons with the potential to kill or seriously injure our child. Most dishwashing detergents include naphta (a central nervous system depressant), diethanolamine (a possible liver poison), and chlorophenylphenol (a metabolic stimulant that is considered a toxic substance).

He states that, of *"all chemicals commonly found in homes, 150 have been linked to allergies, birth defects, cancer, and psychological abnormalities"*.

We have a higher rate of kids with cancer and learning disabilities than ever. If that doesn't say we're doing something wrong in our environment, I'd hate to see what it takes! *According to the American Cancer Society, there has been a 26 percent increase in cancer over the last two decades.*

Dr. Grant also says we should be concerned about the air that our family breathes because *"cleaning products and some personal care products release toxic vapors into the air when they are used and even when they are stored"*. Children may be even more sensitive to chemical fumes. They inhale more air per pound of body weight than adults, and because pollutants are generally heavier than air and collect closer to the floor, small children breathe greater concentrations than grown-ups.

Many people are concerned about the environment, but the environment in our own homes is just as important as outdoors.

If the home care and personal care products we are using are toxic and harmful, we are hurting our families, the environment, and ourselves.

Dr. Grant continues with indoor air pollution as a suspected culprit in sudden infant death syndrome (SIDS). In 1983, a research team at the University of Saskatchewan, Canada, pioneered early research on SIDS and endorphins. SIDS is higher in the winter because of decreased ventilation.

Points to Consider

- The average home today contains sixty-two toxic chemicals, more than a chemistry lab at the turn of the century.

- More than seventy-two thousand synthetic chemicals have been produced since World War II.

- Less than 2 percent of synthetic chemicals have been tested for toxicity, mutagenic, carcinogenic, or birth defects.

- Toxic chemicals in household cleaners are three times more likely to cause cancer than air pollution, and most homes have airborne concentrations of hazardous chemicals that are three to seventy times higher indoors than outdoors.

- Another EPA study stated that the toxic chemicals in household cleaners are three times more likely to cause cancer than outdoor air.

- CMHC reports that houses today are so energy efficient that "outgassing" of chemicals has nowhere to go, so it builds up inside the home.

- We spend 90 percent of our time indoors and 65 percent of our time at home. Moms, infants, and the elderly spend 90 percent of their time in the home.

- The National Cancer Association released results of a fifteen-year study concluding that women who work in the home are at a 54 percent higher risk of developing cancer than women who work outside the home.

- Cancer is the number-one cause of death for children and the number-one killer of women between the ages of thirty-five and fifty-four.

- There has been a call from the US/Canadian Commission to ban bleach in North America. Bleach is being linked to the rising rates of breast cancer in women, reproductive problems in men, and learning and behavioral problems in children.

- There are more than three million poisonings every year. Household cleaners are the number-one cause of poisoning of children.

- Since 1980, asthma has increased by 600 percent. The Canadian Lung Association and the Asthma Society of Canada identify common household cleaners and cosmetics as triggers.

- Formaldehyde, phenol, benzene, toluene, and xylene are found in common household cleaners, cosmetics, beverages, fabrics, and cigarette smoke. These chemicals are carcinogenic and toxic to the immune system.

- There are forty-seven hundred chemicals in tobacco smoke.

In closing, Dr. Grant states that it's important to say that household cleaning and personal care products aren't the only source of chemicals in our home, but they are the easiest ones to replace. What can we do? The answer is to start in small ways at home!

Are you part of the pollution or part of the solution?

According to the US government, the average household is responsible for approximately twenty pounds of toxic waste per year. We can blame big business, but when we put it all together, an average neighborhood of three hundred homes would be adding approximately *six thousand pounds per year to our landfill.*

I live in the southwest corner of Idaho where the population in the four largest cities in the area is approximately 416,000. There are 5,789 subdivisions and 154,000 households.

If every household contributes a minimum of twenty pounds of toxic waste to the landfill per year in my community alone, we would be contributing 3.08 million pounds of toxic waste per year. If you just compare my area with yours, you will see how this problem will grow if we don't become part of the solution rather than continue to be part of the problem.

Most of us would not think of our everyday trash as hazardous, but if you throw away batteries or light bulbs in the trash, you've added toxic chemicals that are going into our soil and water supply.

The following are considered hazardous: oil-based paints, paint thinners, herbicides, insecticides, pesticides, gas, cell phones, computers, batteries, aerosol cans and paints, televisions/electronics, prescriptions, thermometers, household cleaning products, batteries, mercury, motor oil, lawn chemicals, antifreeze, hobby chemicals, fluorescent lights, and any products with warning labels such as "caution" or "keep out of the reach of children."

Here are some tips on what we can do to help:

- Have a special box set aside for the products listed as hazardous, including any household cleaners.

- Don't dump cleaners down the drain or in the water supply.

- Check with your city to see if they provide a place to dispose of hazardous waste items.
  You can make it a family project to collect all hazardous waste and dispose of it properly. Let's all give a hoot and don't pollute. Do the right thing for our planet. Our children's future depends on the decisions we make today.

A new list reveals that we're inundated with hormone disruptors, chemicals that can affect everything from our hearts and our brains to our ability to have babies. I will list the most common household chemicals later in the book.

The development of this list brought to light the fact that hormone-disrupting chemicals that can affect the endocrine glands—pituitary, thyroid, adrenal, thymus, pancreas, ovaries, and testes—can lead to problems with immune systems, bone health, the brain, and heart.

Alf Christophersen quoted on his healthy living blog, *"Just reducing (not eliminating) environmental carcinogens alone would save at least 50,000 lives from cancer annually."*

I am an avid coupon shopper, and I kick myself for all the times that it was more important that I got a "buy one get one free" instead of "buy one that is going to give me peace of mind and is toxin free."

Cynthia Latham, vice president of research and development for the Shaklee Corporation, states the following as part of her company healthy living blog. *"As more toxic chemicals have been introduced to our everyday environment in greater amounts over the last 20 to 30 years, the level of toxins stored in fat cells of our bodies have risen. Bioaccumulation studies have shown that some toxins store in our bodies for life. Greater and greater amounts are being stored at younger ages."*

According to Larry White, author of the February 15, 2011, e-zine article "What's Lurking Under Your Sink," *women who work from home have a 54 percent higher death rate from cancer than women who work outside of the home."* The higher death rate is believed to be due to daily exposure to chemicals found in ordinary household products.

As a hypnotherapist, a mother, a grandmother, an entrepreneur who has had a home-based business since 1975, and a two-time cancer survivor, I should be asking myself "Why? Why am I still here?" I remember a particular close call in February 1998 when I had a very restless night one Saturday and didn't sleep because of a pain in the upper part of my right leg. I went to the hospital for an x- ray to see if there was a problem, and soon the radiologist walked in and said he couldn't find anything wrong with my leg.

What a relief. But his next statement wasn't as reassuring when he said, "You need to find a doctor right away because you have a large tumor on each ovary." That completely shocked me because I didn't know I had ovaries; I'd had a complete hysterectomy when I was twenty-six years old, over twenty years earlier. Within a week, I found a doctor and had surgery. The ovaries and tumors were removed in the nick of time. It required a colon surgeon and gynecologist to complete the surgery because the tumors were attached to the colon wall and my stomach. It was a miracle that the radiologist had found the tumors.

You probably know someone close to you who has had cancer. It may have been a coworker, neighbor, friend, or family member. The list could keep going. In hypnotherapy, I share with my clients that long-term anger, pain, and hostility trigger cancer and heart problems. You may ask how that is possible, and I would respond that all three are toxic emotions, which are as dangerous as toxic chemicals that enter the human body. It is important that we understand the direct correlation between our thoughts and our physical health.

Our subconscious mind hears our thoughts and will respond accordingly. Its function is to either help you thrive or to protect you from dangers, real or imagined. We are in a constant state of emotional stress. We are rushing around. We are bombarded with news. We are fighting traffic and are stressed out at work or home. And so forth.

When does our body have time to decompress? When this continues day after day, week after week, it is no wonder that we have so much illness and disease in our society. When people are under stress, they oftentimes turn to the use of antidepressants, alcohol and drugs, and sleep aids, which only adds to your problems. But the beauty is that it can all be changed because it is only a perception, and perceptions can be changed.

Toxic-free living is a choice. It starts with choosing toxic-free cleaning, skin, and body products, trying to buy more organic foods, and shopping the perimeter of the store instead of the center aisles. Then of course, surround yourself with friends who enhance you and bring out the best that is in you. If your friends don't make you feel good about who you are, you need to love them and release them. You deserve to feel good about yourself.

This is why understanding how our thoughts, feelings, and emotions are vital to not only our emotional well-being but our physical health is so important. If we live in fear, anger, hurt, or any other negative emotional state, our physical body is affected on a cellular level as well. Changing our perception of any given situation is key to altering the pattern of our life.

When we find ourselves in a toxic environment or experience negativity, we may consciously tell ourselves that we can control the situation and be fine. But if we do not believe we are safe, our cells will respond accordingly. If this belief continues for a long period of time, the cells and DNA will adapt and change according to the perception of the subconscious images.

These changes eventually manifest as physical and mental disease in the body. As signals are sent from the environment, positive or negative, your cells will respond.

I took advanced Hypnotherapy training in Florida. My trainer was sharing his story about being in the middle of a hypnosis session one day when he had a massive heart attack. He told about his thoughts as the ambulance was racing toward the hospital.

I abruptly asked him, "If long-term anger, pain, and hostility can cause heart attacks and cancer, which was it with you?"

He promptly said, "Anger."
I then asked, "What did you do about it?"
He immediately said, "I decided it was time to release it and let it go."
Considering his other options, it was a wise choice, don't you think?
What messages are you sending your body on a daily basis? Are you sending healthy, happy messages or mixed signals?

Lessons I've Learned in My Life!

Always trust your intuition. If you can't hear it, you have too much clutter in your life. Take ten minutes each day to sit quietly. Close your eyes. If you breathe deep and softly, you will start to hear your inner voice. Over time, you will learn to listen to your intuition, and you will soon realize it is always right.

Chapter 2 Review

1. Check all that apply. Household chemicals have been linked to:

   Birth Defects   Psychological Abnormalities

   Allergies   Childhood Cancer

   Cancer stay-at-home moms,   Sudden Infant Death Syndrome

   Learning Disabilities,   or all of the above.

2. Check all that apply: Which of the following products are considered toxic:

Prescriptions	Hobby Paints,	Cell Phones	Thermometers
Batteries,	Clorox,	Fluoride	Fluorescent Bulbs
toothpaste,	Aerosol Containers,	Ajax,	or all of the above.

Janet Starr Hull is an OSHA-certified environmental hazardous waste emergency response specialist and toxicologist. In 1991, Dr. Hull had an unexpected change in career after she was diagnosed with incurable Graves' disease. Through diligent research and her thorough understanding of toxicity, she later discovered her disease was actually aspartame poisoning. For more about Dr. Hull or to receive her free newsletter, you can go to her website at www.janethull.com.

Many of us have no idea if we are exposed to toxic chemicals. Pay close attention to the products you are using in and around your home, including body and hair care products. Removing toxic chemicals from your household environment can make a huge difference if done as soon as symptoms become a chronic concern. Dr. Starr compiled the following A–Z symptoms of chemical toxicity.

Allergies.	Angina.	Colitis
Birth defects	Brain Damage	Dizziness/Vertigo
Fibromyalgia	ADD/ADHD	Impulsiveness/OCD

Anemia	Lung damage	Neurological disorders
Skin ailments/rashes	Constipation	Breathing problems
Dry skin/eyes	Loss of hair	Loss of memory
Metabolic problems	Seizures	Tumors
Blurred vision	Depression	Loss of libido
Headaches/Migraines	Lung damage.	Indigestion/Acid Reflux
Skeletal malformation	Nerve disorders	Vitamin deficiencies
Insomnia.	Cataracts.	Behavioral Changes.
Fatigue.	Eye Damage	

Common symptoms of chemical toxicity A–Z

3. Check the answer that applies. If you told your friend a secret, she would:

   - Keep your confidence forever.
   - Try to keep it a secret but might slip it out by accident.
   - Share it with others immediately.

4. Check the answer that applies. If you had a problem, you would:

   - Tell your friend you had a problem but didn't want to share it.
   - Say nothing because you remember how it backfired the last time you spoke to her about a problem you were having.
   - Share it with your friend and seek her advice.

5. Check the answer that applies. If you wanted to get together with your friend but she had a prior commitment, she would most likely:

   - Apologize for being unavailable and set a specific time to get together.
   - If appropriate, ask you if you'd like to come along.
   - Go into detail about her busy schedule.

6. Check the answer that applies. When you call your friend, she usually:

    *   Takes your call as long as it's feasible to put aside what she is doing.
    *   Tells you she's really busy but will try to call you back.
    *   Tells you she's busy and you should call her back another time.

7. Check the answer that applies. When you and your friend go to the movies:

    *   You discuss the movie you'd both like to see.
    *   Your friend will often pick the movie but will ask if you agree.
    *   Your friend always has to pick the movie even if you have very different suggestions.

8. Check the answer that applies. The best thing you can say about this particular friend is that she:

    *   Enjoys doing the same things you do.
    *   Shares your values and beliefs and cares about you.
    *   Can get you complimentary tickets to the hottest concerts.

9. Check the answer that applies. If your friend made a mistake that affected you, she would most likely:

    *   Ignore the situation.
    *   Apologize to you and ask your forgiveness.
    *   Blame you even if it were her fault.

10. Check the answer that applies. If a few weeks went by and your friend hadn't heard from you, she would probably:

    *   Wait as long as it took for you to call or contact her. You're always the one to initiate communication.
    *   Send you an e-mail or call you to find out how you're doing.

- Call and interrogate you about why you hadn't contacted her sooner.

Is Your Friend Toxic?

Pay attention when your friend puts you down. Be wary of a friend who gossips about you. Consider mockery carefully. Consider your feelings about your friend and the time spent together. Ask yourself these questions:

- Is this something that your friend has just started to do, or has it been going on for a long time?
- Does spending time with your friend make you feel defensive or upset?
- Do you spend time justifying your own behavior around your friend instead of it feeling natural to be together?
- Do you feel belittled, attacked, or used? Does the friendship feel unbalanced and like plain hard work?
- Do you feel at fault for things that happen to your friend?
- Has your friend betrayed your confidences?
- Does it feel like competition rather than a balanced and caring friendship?

If you answered yes to any of the above questions, your friendship is toxic for both of you. Sometimes the best solution to toxic relationships is to love them but release them.

Lessons I've Learned in My Life!

Keep people in your life who truly love you, motivate you, encourage you, enhance you, and make you happy. If you know people who do none of these things, let them go.

3

CHEMICALS EXPOSED

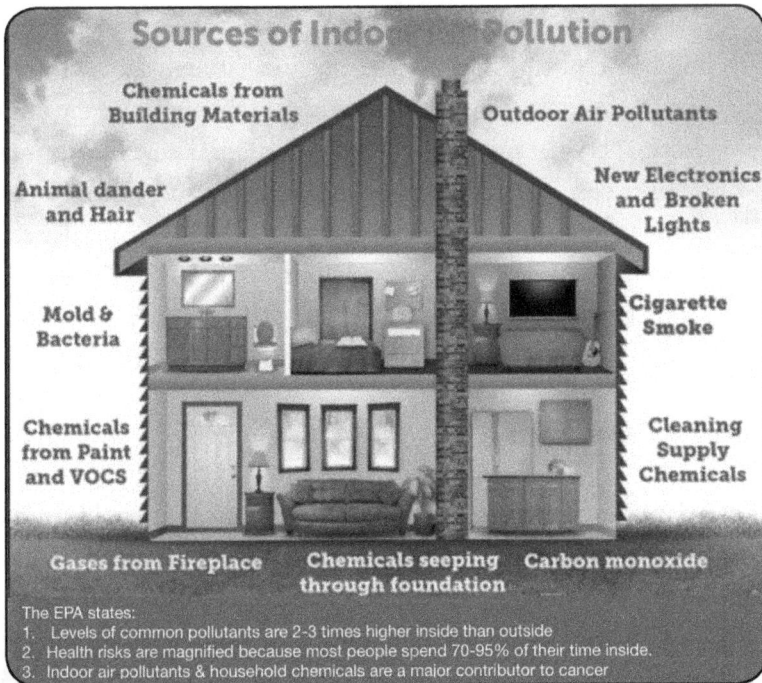

Sources of Indoor Air Pollution

Chemicals from Building Materials

Outdoor Air Pollutants

Animal dander and Hair

New Electronics and Broken Lights

Mold & Bacteria

Cigarette Smoke

Chemicals from Paint and VOCS

Cleaning Supply Chemicals

Gases from Fireplace   Chemicals seeping   Carbon monoxide
through foundation

The EPA states:
1. Levels of common pollutants are 2-3 times higher inside than outside
2. Health risks are magnified because most people spend 70-95% of their time inside.
3. Indoor air pollutants & household chemicals are a major contributor to cancer

We are getting exposure to toxins via swallowing (ingestion), breathing (inhalation), or skin or eyes (absorption). Daily exposure to common toxins includes:

- exhaust fumes
- air pollution—for example, working in or around chemicals in the home, workplace, and outside
- pesticides, herbicides, and fertilizers in food and water

- animal products containing hormones, antibiotics, and parasite treatments
- drugs, prescribed and recreational—for example, alcohol, & tobacco,
- additives in food—for example, colorings, flavorings, and preservatives
- carcinogenic ingredients in personal care and cleaning products
- off-gassing of furniture, appliances, paints, and so forth
- electromagnetic radiation (EMRs)

  We know that the personal care products we put on our skin and hair create possible toxic exposures through skin absorption, but do we really realize how many toxic chemicals we are talking about and what products we are including? These include soaps, lotions, cosmetics, shampoos, deodorants, and other common products. The list could go on and on. Of 2,983 chemicals used in personal care products, 884 were found to be toxic, 778 can cause acute toxicity, 146 can cause tumors, 218 can cause reproductive complications, and 376 can cause skin and eye irritations.

Death by Detergent

Sometimes we don't stop to think how dangerous household products that we store under our kitchen cabinet can be when combined. I have a friend who grabbed a bottle of hydrogen peroxide to use in an experiment. He had a diluted bottle and a full-strength bottle, but he had planned on using the diluted bottle. In his haste, he grabbed the full- strength bottle and drank a portion of it, and he immediately realized his mistake. He almost died, and he was paralyzed for months and then graduated to wearing leg braces. He was lucky and survived, but his recovery process was very slow so we must never forget that household chemicals can be just as deadly as some of the most powerful drugs on the market if they are used improperly or placed in the wrong hands.

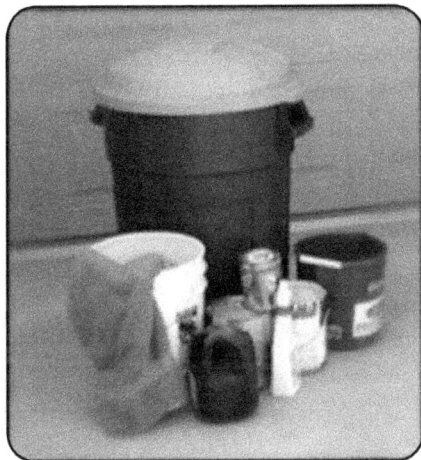

Susan was a newlywed of twenty-one. She put several household chemicals in the bathtub at once, hoping to please her husband with a shiny tub. It happened to be during the early winter days when there was frost on the windows so she left the bathroom window closed to keep the room warm.

Within minutes, she felt very queasy and light-headed and almost passed out. It was a scary experience that almost killed her. She didn't realize that the simple mixture of common household cleaners could become both a toxic and deadly combination. It's another reason to think about going green and using toxic-free products.

I want to make sure everybody knows the dangers of what can happen when you mix common household cleaning products.

Chapter 3 Review

1. How are toxic chemicals entering our body?

   _____

   _____

   _____

2. What are at least four common ways we are getting exposed to toxic chemicals daily?

   _____

   _____

   _____

3. Susan mixed common household cleaners when she cleaned her bathtub. Is it safe to mix your household cleaners together?

   _____

   _____

   _____

4. Is your home chemical free or a danger zone?

   _____

   _____

   _____

Lessons I've Learned in My Life!

- A bad mistake becomes a good lesson if you learn from it, but you can't make the same mistake twice. The second time you make it, it's no longer a mistake. It's a choice.

- It is best to give advice in only two circumstances: when it is requested and when it is a life-threatening situation.

4

WHO IS AT RISK?

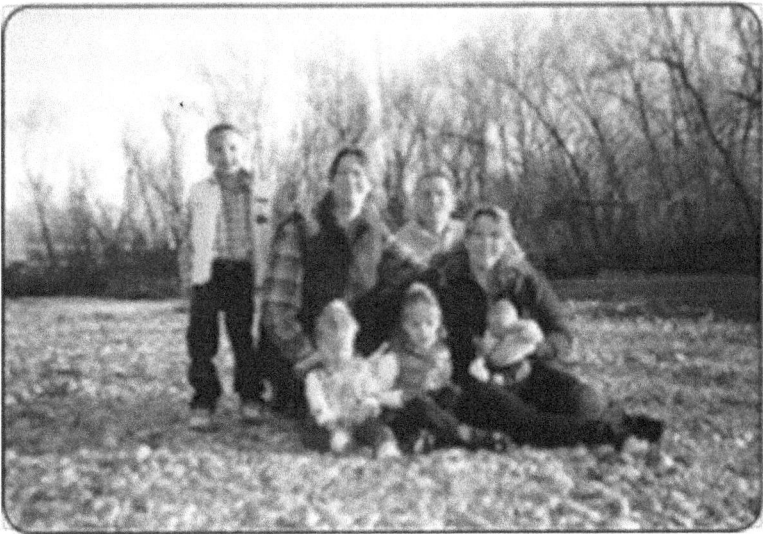

Our family homes are chemical-free.
We have learned it is better to be safe than sorry.

My son and his family...... introduced me to toxic-free products.

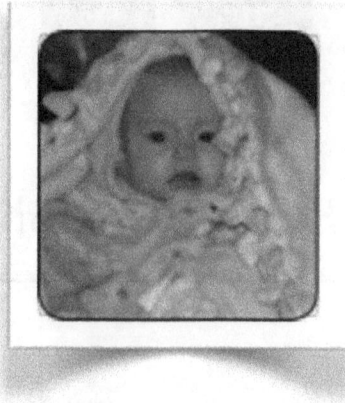

Children and pets have a greater risk
of exposure to toxic chemicals.

Children are always so curious that they are getting into everything and have absolutely no conception of dangerous or harmful. As a parent or grandparent, you should always be on high alert when it is quiet. That is when you know they are up to no good.

My four-year-old granddaughter decided she wanted to paint her fingernails, toenails, and the white carpet with hot-pink nail polish without telling anyone. One month later, her mom discovered the mishap behind the furniture, and by this time, it looked like it was permanently in place. She didn't want to use any harsh chemicals around the children or the pets. My daughter-in-law was sharing her frustration with the karate teacher, and he gave her a toxic-free product from a local manufacturer to take home. It removed the polish immediately. What I thought was commendable was that she would have kept her hot-pink carpet before exposing her precious children to toxic chemicals.

According to www.greencleancertified.com, the most common methods of exposure are through the skin and respiratory tract. Children are frequently in contact with the chemical residue that housecleaning products leave behind by crawling, lying, and sitting on the freshly cleaned floor.

Children, especially infants and toddlers, frequently put their fingers in their mouths and noses, increasing risks for exposure. When infants start to eat solid food, it is common that food is placed directly on a high chair tray that has just been wiped down with a household cleaner or dish detergent.

Another factor is that children's exposure rate is much higher because, even though the amount of chemicals they are exposed to remains equal, children's bodies are smaller so the concentration is stronger; plus, their immune systems are still developing.

For many of the same reasons, pets are also at risk. They are low to the ground, they lick their paws, and they are close enough to eat food from the table and floor. They are nosy enough to stick their nose and mouth in the dishwashing dispenser of the open door on the dishwasher or drink out of the toilet bowl and wherever else they decide.

RON AND TAFFY AND THEIR FAVORITE PASTIME

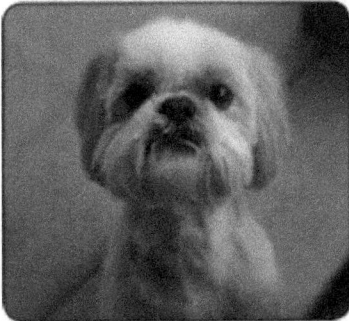

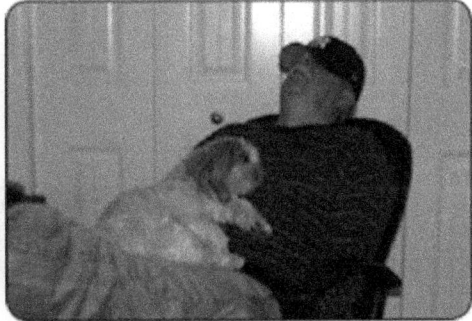

This is my nosy little Taffy, the most adorable little shih tzu. She was one and a half when she came to live with us, and she was absolutely the most perfect little lapdog in the world. She was supposed to be my lapdog, but my husband had no life, so she stayed glued to his lap. She would lie on his head, chest, neck, back, and so forth. Anytime she saw him start to sit, she ran as fast as she could and flew into the air and landed on him. We only had her for two short years when she suddenly stopped eating and was sleeping a lot, and when she did get up, she started walking in circles. The doctor said her liver enzyme was over six hundred, and they thought she probably got into something toxic and her little system couldn't handle it. She died, and my husband and I were total basket cases. I still cry when I look at her pictures because she was so much fun. It is so easy for pets to get into toxic products, and their systems cannot handle the chemicals, but we keep everything down at their level where they can sniff and lick.

Next on the list of vulnerability are people who have had cancer in the past, closely followed by people with compromised immune systems.

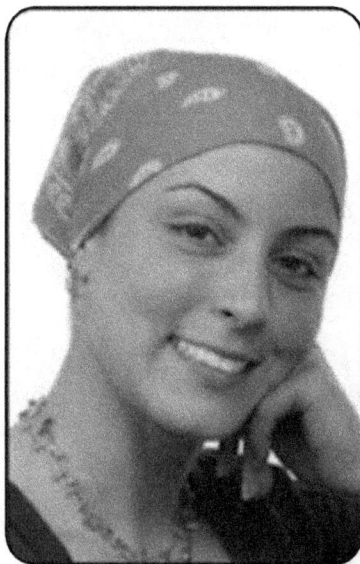

The elderly would be considered our next at-risk group due to the fact they sometimes have health challenges and compromised immune systems as well.

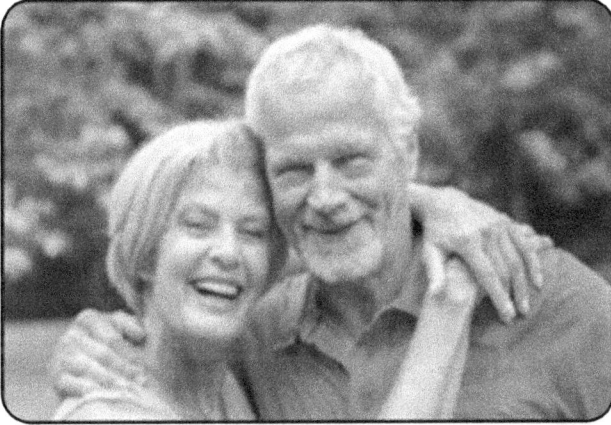

Repeated Exposure

You may be thinking that the diluted aspect of off-the-shelf cleaning products reduces or all together eliminates the threat of getting sick from your floor polish, window cleaner, or air freshener. However, many of the toxins found in these products (and other cleaning products) are bio-accumulative, meaning the chemicals do not purge easily from the body, and over time, even mild exposures can add up to toxic levels. In fact, a medical study recently conducted in Iowa suggests a correlation between certain occupations and bladder cancer. One of those occupations is cleaning services.

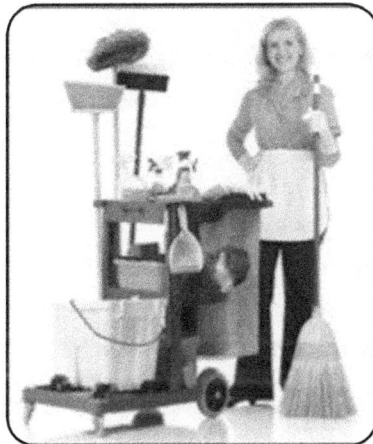

These products are used repeatedly and routinely in the home to maintain cleanliness, increasing the chances for bioaccumulation of chemicals in the body

When we read a story, we usually think *that is so sad but it could never happen to me*, but it can. I remember the days of coupon shopping when I chose cheap instead of reading the label to see if there were warning labels or known toxic chemicals.

I would like to share another story of a doctor who also found out how deadly just a few toxins can be on the human body. Lisa wrote this article for the *Women's Health Activist* newsletter in 2009 and gave me permission to share it with you. Since that time, she now dedicates her medical practice to environmental health in Vineyard Haven, Massachusetts.

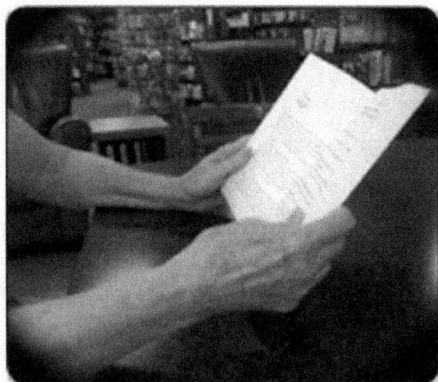

Environmental toxins can cause medical problems that are difficult for the average doctor to identify and treat. The more severe "environmental illnesses" include chemical sensitivity, chronic fatigue syndrome (CFS), fibromyalgia, and Gulf War syndrome. Milder, environmentally induced illnesses are all around us and include anxiety, allergies, autoimmunity, and intolerances to chemicals. The toxins found in pesticides, solvents,

heavy metals, and especially those produced by indoor mold can hit women especially hard.

Women are four times more likely to exhibit symptoms of chronic fatigue syndrome and chemical sensitivity than men are. Worse, it can be overwhelming for people (particularly those who are already ill) to learn about living a less toxic lifestyle and avoiding environmental contaminants. Environmental medicine offers specific answers by giving both doctors and patients the tools to treat illnesses caused by toxic exposures. Sadly, very few people learn about environmental medicine until they are on death's door, as I was.

In 2001, a muscle biopsy showed my cells lacked oxygen, and I was told I was dying from something resembling Amyotrophic Lateral Sclerosis (ALS, often called Lou Gehrig's disease). My facial muscles couldn't produce a smile, and I gasped for air all night. I was so weak I could no longer fold a towel or wash my hair.

Eventually, my husband, dog, and I all developed adrenal failure as well. I was very fortunate to get connected to the Environmental Health Center of Dallas and to recover. Our household illnesses were caused by mold found in the huge aquarium shed attached to my home, which produced dangerous mycotoxins called "trichothecenes."

Trichothecenes are commonly found in the urine of sick people living in moldy homes. These toxins are used as bioterrorism agents and have been extensively studied by the Army. The Army has found that female rats exposed to airborne trichothecenes develop adrenal necrosis (death of the gland that makes steroid hormones). In humans, adrenal insufficiency causes health problems, including depression, fatigue, allergies, low blood pressure, dizziness on standing, anxiety, intolerance of stress, hypoglycemia, weight loss, tearfulness, and increased sense of smell.

These are symptoms of environmental illness often found in women who live in moldy homes, like I did. The Army's research shows that testosterone may help protect men from toxins such as trichothecenes, which could explain why men are less likely to develop the same symptoms as women.

A sizable proportion of the US population suffers, often unknowingly, from environmental illnesses. About 15 percent of the population has been told by a doctor they are chemically sensitive, and about 5 percent is disabled by the condition and cannot be exposed to chemicals such as those found in air fresheners, perfume, and smoke. Fully 30 percent of elderly and CFS patients are chemically sensitive. Yet few doctors have learned about chemical sensitivity or chronic fatigue or learned how they can be treated with environmental medicine.

In my many years of medical training, I never even heard of these environmental illnesses. That's because the symptoms of environmental illness are not included in either medical school curricula or residency training. To this day, the American Medical Association's (AMA) eighteen-year-old policy is that environmental medicine lacks substantiating data and that environmental illness (EI) and chronic fatigue are not valid diagnoses. My organization is working now to change that policy.

The American Academy of Environmental Medicine trains physicians to assess all potential causes of ill health. The term "environmental illnesses" describes these conditions' unifying symptoms, as well as hormonal, neurotransmitter, nutritional, and genetic abnormalities that cause disease. A recent study examined cerebrospinal fluid proteins in patients suffering from Gulf War syndrome, chronic fatigue syndrome, and fibromyalgia, many of whom also showed symptoms of chemical sensitivity. The study " found a unique set of proteins" in these patients' cerebrospinal fluid. The author suggests that, "although the syndrome names are different, the presumed pathologic mechanisms may be shared." Environmental medicine practitioners also suspect that environmental factors affect diseases including Parkinson's disease, multiple sclerosis, ALS, autoimmune diseases, autism, and attention- deficit/hyperactivity disorder (ADHD).

The need to understand environmental exposure is particularly essential for women with cancer. Research indicates that mold toxins and pesticides can cause cancers, including breast and uterine cancer.

There is even a test for trichothecenes in food that indicates that it increases DNA transcription in breast cancer cells. This could mean that living in a moldy home may increase the growth of existing breast cancer. Avoidance of potentially dangerous chemicals, including bisphenol A (BPA) and phthalates, commonly used industrial compounds that are often found in plastic containers and food cans, would be wise as well.

I firmly believe that one reason that environmental illnesses are not taken more seriously is because it is chiefly women who develop them. Many women experience cognitive and mental health problems along with environmental illness. When they go to the doctor, they may suffer from mental or cognitive impairment, but their behavior actually results from being environmentally ill. Too often, physicians focus on women's mental health symptoms and insultingly recommend psychiatry when these patients actually need an environmental medicine specialist. When toxicity is treated, mental and physical symptoms can dramatically improve or disappear.

As a result of my horrific personal experience, I founded the Preventive and Environmental Health Alliance to advance clinical and public awareness of environmental illnesses. Women have to know about environmental illness. The AMA needs to change its stance and promote a sanctioned specialty (Environmental and Integrative Medicine) to train doctors to correctly identify these diseases. Insurance companies need to expand reimbursement for allergy testing, nutritional assessments, and effective treatments.

*More research is needed on detoxification treatments that work, such as sauna, **thermotherapy with the BioMat,** intravenous vitamins, oxygen therapy, chelation, immune modification, hormone replacement, and antigen therapy.*

This is the preventive medicine of the future. If you are concerned about exposure, I encourage you to get involved! Help us to push for congressional support for environmental health legislation. No one should suffer alone from these conditions.

Women suffering from environmental illnesses do not need drugs and condescension; they need referral and information from better-informed doctors! We must insist on being heard; we must help the millions of women, our sisters, who are too ill to help themselves. We must work together and present a unified force to demand a greater focus on this women's health issue, right now.

Lisa Nagy, MD, was appointed to the Centers for Disease Control and Prevention's (CDC) Working Group on the Scientific Understanding of the Effect of Chemicals on Human Health. She is also the founder and president of the Preventive and Environmental Health Alliance. The story of Lisa and her family will soon be made into a movie. A new book is in the works,

How to Be a Better Doctor: Believe the Patient. http://green.wikia.com/ wiki/ Toxins in Household Cleaning Products

Chapter 4 Review

1. Which are the four categories of people at the greatest risk for exposure from toxic chemicals in household cleaning products?

   _____.   _____

   _____.   _____

2. What does it mean when a toxic chemical is bio-accumulative?

   _____

   _____

   _____

3. What toxin was Dr. Lisa Nagy and her family exposed to in 2001 that caused her devastating illness?

   _____

   _____

   _____

4. Eventually, Dr. Lisa was able to find a doctor who was able to diagnose, treat, and help her heal from a very long illness. What type of doctor did she find?

   _____

   _____

   _____

Lessons I've Learned in My Life!

A great outfit doesn't mean much when you feel like total dog poop. Great health means more than high heels and manicured nails.

5

BEHIND ENEMY LINES!

H ow are the household chemicals you assume are safe affecting your health? I was very fortunate to meet Dr. Mike McCullough a few years ago, and he has been my mentor ever since. If I have any questions about nutrition, toxic chemicals, or health concerns, Dr. McCullough is always the first person I think to call because he is an encyclopedia of knowledge. Here is Dr. Mike's personal journey as he discovered firsthand the role that toxic chemicals can play in causing health problems.

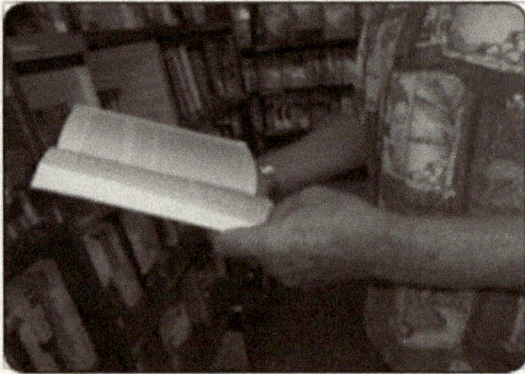

I have been involved in health issues as far back as high school. I remember having excessive bleeding from the age of nine until I was in high school. At that young age, I knew there was something wrong with my body so I started looking at natural ingredients and products. Other than the constant nose bleeds, I have been interested in exercise and health so chiropractic was a natural progression for me.

Another thing that came into play over the years was my family history, which also was a contributing factor in my belief that, if I were going to live a long and healthy life, I needed to pay more attention to what I was using on and in my body.

My dad had a quadruple heart bypass surgery at the age of forty-six, my mother died of colon cancer at age sixty-one, my dad's five brothers had some form of heart disease before the age of fifty, my oldest brother's son died from a heart attack at age thirty-nine, and my brother, who was a year younger than I am, died of a heart attack in 2010.

When I was in high school, I worked as a painter in a union for two local painting contractors. At the time, I didn't realize how caustic and damaging the paint was that we were using. Some of it was latex, and some of it was oil-based. As an apprentice, my job was to wash the brushes for all of the painters. We never used protective gloves to wash the brushes and painting equipment because we didn't realize how dangerous chemicals could be absorbed through the skin and go directly to the bloodstream.

In the late sixties and early seventies, ammonia was used to make some latex paints. I can remember pulling out globs of latex paint from the corner of my eyes after spray painting, even after wearing protective goggles.

At that time, I didn't realize it was the effects of the chemicals in the paint that was making me sick and rundown.

Years later in chiropractic school, I would occasionally help my neighbor, who was a painting contractor, on the weekends. Whenever I would paint the inside of buildings, I would get violently sick and didn't realize the fumes from the paint were affecting me.

I finally connected the problem with chemical sensitivities while in chiropractic school after becoming ill during cadaver dissections. The cadavers we used were embalmed with formaldehyde, and we would spend two to three hours a day in the dissection labs.

What solidified my speculations on the chemical sensitivity resulted from my trips to the Laundromat. I would use various name-brand laundry detergents sold in the vending machines to wash my clothes and sheets. The first few days after going to the Laundromat, I always felt sick and had difficulty concentrating at school.

In my senior year of chiropractic school, we had a course in toxic chemicals that helped put my chemical sensitivity problem together. Now I could predict when I would feel sick and what caused it.

After graduating from school in 1985, I returned to Boise, Idaho, to practice. In 1988, I was introduced to a natural-based consumer manufacturing company that developed a brand of environmentally safe home cleaning products that have made a world of difference in the way I felt, and my health improved dramatically.

Q&A: Judie Dietzler and Dr. McCullough

Have you seen any research about how toxins in household products affect the health of consumers?

- *There is a vast amount of research concerning household chemicals and their negative effects. The EPA does not regulate household chemicals to the extent of regulations on commercially used chemicals. All we have to do is look on the labels and read, and it will tell us how unsafe the products are. If people ask me what I can do to improve my health, the first thing I tell them is to clean up the toxins in their house to get rid of the free radicals that cause cancer. The chemicals in your home are outgassing, just like the sealed cleaning products at the grocery store, and if you want to see a noticeable improvement in your health, you need to improve the environment in your home. If you take vitamins, that's your business, but what you put down your drain is our business. Most water treatment plants are unable to remove phosphates, disinfectants, hormones, and other harsh chemicals.*

What would be one key advice you would give consumers about chemicals in their household products?

- *I hope I have been able to help readers understand how dangerous they are and the damage that chemicals are causing to both their families and the environment. The government is not looking out for our safety. If they would only read the labels and ask themselves, "Why am I so loyal to this manufacturer when there are safer, more effective natural products available at a lesser cost?"*

How Exposure to Cleaning Products Can Affect Our Health

You may think that you can dilute off-the-shelf cleaning products with water to eliminate the threat of getting sick from your floor polish, window cleaner, or air freshener. However, many of the toxins found in these products (and so many other cleaning products) are bio-accumulative, meaning the chemicals do not purge easily from the body, and over time, even mild exposures can add up to toxic levels.

Research points to the toxic effects of not only active but also inactive ingredients of household cleaning products plus body and hair care items that can affect the central nervous, reproductive, and neurological systems through your skin by breathing and ingesting.

The following is a description of how toxic chemicals affect you in each of three essential categories:

Carcinogens

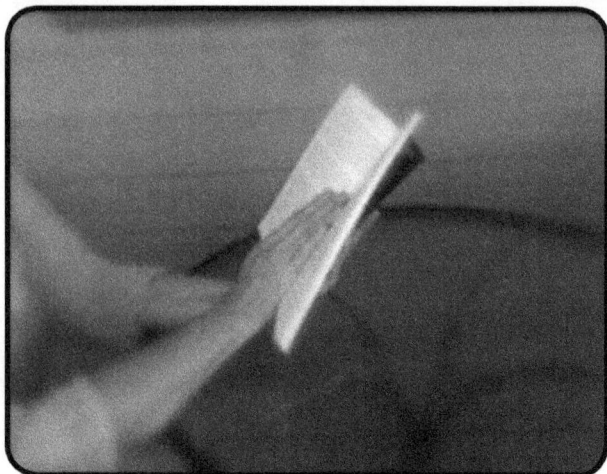

Carcinogens cause cancer and/or promote cancer's growth. A women's risk of breast cancer (US) in the 1940s was one in twenty-two. In 2004, it was one in seven. Why? Breast cancer is the leading cause of death in women ages thirty-four to forty-four. The first health effects of environmental toxins causing cancer were seen in the early 1900s.

What causes cancer? There are internal factors like hormones and immune or inherited conditions. Then there are external factors like lifestyle habits (smoking, diet, and alcohol), viruses, chemicals, and radiation.

Sometimes our choices to have a toxin enter our life may be because of a crisis, and we may not have the time or energy to make the healthier choice because we don't have all of the facts. Over the years, I have had many clients walk through my door due to an array of problems ranging from smoking, weight loss, stuttering, motivation, and/or pain control, but several years ago, a number of my clients were breast implant survivors. They were a variety of ages with symptoms that would range from bone and joint pain to neurological problems. The one thing they all had in common was that they were very sick women.

The word *cancer* can be frightening, but when you follow it up with *mastectomy*, that can be total devastation to many women. That is why I am so passionate about making sure they know all of the facts about breast implants before they decide implants will make them whole again.

Some women get ill immediately; some may take longer. I believe all will feel the effects of breast implants from either mold, fungus, or silicone damaging their joints, brain, blood vessels, cells, muscles, or tissues at some point during their lives.

You will find a list of the pros and cons of breast implants in the book *The Naked Truth about Breast Implants* (Lighthouse Publishing, 2009), and a list of the toxic chemicals in the implants. Then you are able to make an informed decision.

I would like to share a toxic story of a saline breast implant recipient whom we will call Mary for the sake of her identity. According to plastic surgeons and the manufacturers, saline implants are the "safe" implants.

In the fall of 2005, she was diagnosed with stage two breast cancer and had a modified radical mastectomy. The doctors determined that she was at high risk for a second primary tumor in the other breast so the final decision was a double mastectomy. She was interested in having a flap surgery using her own tissue, but because there wasn't any surgeon versed in doing a free-flap in her state at that time, she wasn't opposed to having implants because she was assured they were safe. Her plastic surgeon advised her that, if there were any problems, it would be easier to remove the implants than it would be to correct a problem with flap surgery.

She opted for saline-filled implants because, by then, there was some talk of silicone gel-filled implants leaking. A Mentor saline implant was surgically implanted in her chest cavity in October 2005. But in less than a month, she suddenly became ill with symptoms of widespread joint and muscle pain, stomach cramps and diarrhea, fatigue, hair loss, and morning stiffness so severe that she could barely get out of bed.

One day, she did a Google search and discovered for the first time that the shells of her saline implants were made of silicone. She decided that she wanted the implants out, but the doctor refused. It was another nine months before she found a doctor who could remove her implants, and by that time, her consulting business was almost at a standstill.

The implants were out, but the health problems continued. The pain was unrelenting and at times so excruciating that she was bedridden and disoriented. Her doctors had no idea what was wrong, but she was eventually diagnosed with fibromyalgia, given medication for pain, and sent home. The medication made her so drowsy that she could barely stay awake at work. She had continual pain and memory loss that made it hard for her to remember all of the work details so she finally closed her consulting business.

In 2008, she learned that, in order to ensure maximum removal of the silicone from the shell, the scar tissue capsules had to be removed. Unfortunately, her capsules had not been removed. Because the capsules are located under her muscles, she was told that removing them now could do more harm than good. There wasn't a guarantee that they could be removed fully intact. There was a possibility that the doctors would have to scrape the capsules off her ribs.

She developed a sleep disorder and tried a number of medications, and the doctor prescribed her Ambien for sleep, which caused a whole new set of problems and added additional toxins that she didn't need. She had fibromyalgia, IBS, Raynaud's, and cognitive memory problems. Her marriage ended in divorce, she was placed on disability, and she had to move in with her parents. Not exactly what she dreamed of as her fairy tale life.

She would have been so much better and healthier if she'd had the double mastectomy and a special-fitted bra and said no to the implants. She would have looked in the mirror, and a beautiful woman would have been looking back at her. She should be a cancer survivor, not a cancer survivor who had to then go on and live with and survive breast implant illnesses. After all, a foreign material is a foreign material.

I am reminded of a dear friend several years ago who was so excited when she got saline breast implants. She couldn't actually afford them, so her boyfriend paid for them, and her outward self-esteem soared. But after three or four years, she started having health issues, fatigue, and joint pains. Then suddenly, one breast implant deflated. She no longer had the boyfriend, and she didn't have the money to replace the implant.

Her health took a severe turn for the worse so she finally went to the doctor and discovered she had an inoperable brain tumor. She lost her job at the printing company and had to keep moving into less expensive apartments. I am not sure what happened to her, but I think of her often as I remember her initial enthusiasm and the devastation that followed.

Toxic chemicals are part of our life in many different forms. Sometimes:

- You can't see the toxins unless you are in Los Angeles when it's smoggy.

- You hear them when someone is shouting cruel, hurtful words your way.

- You feel the toxins when bleach is splashed in your eyes.

But there are also times when you may believe doctors and the government when they say a product is safe instead of researching and listening to your own inner voice of wisdom and common sense. That is why I included the stories about breast implants. I believe there will be a point in time that there will be as great a controversy over breast implants as there was over cigarette smoking. It will take longer because it is a women's issue, but it will happen. Saline implants are not a safer alternative to silicone.

- Symptoms of breast implant sickness include cognitive dysfunction (short-term memory loss), swollen lymph glands, Sjogren's syndrome (dryness in the mouth, kidneys, eyes, and lungs), scleroderma, rheumatoid arthritis, severe joint and muscle pain, incapacitating fatigue, multiple allergies, headaches, peripheral numbness, hair loss, central nervous system disorders (similar to multiple sclerosis), and silicosis (a respiratory lung disease).

Chemicals in Breast Implants

Polyvinyl Chloride (Liquid Vinyl)	Urethane	Lacquer Thinner
Dichlorometha	Epoxy Resin	Epoxy Hardener
Amine	Printing Ink	Toluene
Acetone	Formaldehyde	Talcum Powder
Metal cleaning acid	Color Pigments	Oakite
Eastman 910-glue	Ethylene Oxide	Carbon Black
Xylene	Hexone	Thixon-OSN-2

Rubber	Acid stearic	Zinc Oxide
Rubber Solvent	Phenol	Benzene
Methyl Ethyl Ketone	Cyclohexanone	Isopropyl Alcohol

People working in the plants that manufacture these chemicals even limit their exposure to them. It's unbelievable that we put this stuff in our bodies. These are only a few of the thirty- eight chemicals found in implants. Now just imagine what happens if the implants rupture. Better pray that they won't!

There are no less than seven solvents in breast implants and a minimum of four known carcinogens, and silicone benzene is known to depress the immune system and can cause leukemia.

Plus, *there are well over a dozen toxic chemicals.* Once you know all of the facts and you talk to hundreds of sick women like I have, it is hard to imagine why anyone would choose to go down this road, but they do every day.

Endocrine Disruptors

Endocrine disruptors mimic human hormones, confusing the body with false signals. Exposure to endocrine disruptors can lead to numerous health concerns, including reproductive, developmental, growth, and behavior problems. Endocrine disruptors have been linked to reduced fertility, premature puberty, miscarriage, menstrual problems, challenged immune systems, abnormal prostate size, ADHD, non-Hodgkin's lymphoma, and cancer.

In the 1940s and 1950s, the chemical industry discovered that BPA was an excellent hardener for epoxy resins and plastic polycarbonate. There is an estimated six billion pounds used in consumer products per year with low-dose effects on the endocrine system.

The endocrine system is one of the body's main systems for controlling and coordinating the body's work. It produces hormones, chemical messages that travel through the blood to specific parts of the body where they help maintain all tissues and organ systems. Hormones control some of the following actions: body energy levels, reproduction, growth and sexual development, internal balance of body systems, responses to stress and injury, and bone and muscle strength.

Endocrine glands and endocrine-related organs are like factories. They produce and store hormones and release them as needed. When the body needs these substances, the bloodstream carries the proper types of hormones to specific targets. These targets may be organs, tissues, or cells.

Hormone-excreting glands include the pineal, pituitary, thyroid, and adrenal glands, along with the pancreas, ovary, and testes. The following chart shows the gland and the function of the gland:

Gland (location)	Example hormone	Function
Pineal gland (brain)	Melatonin	Sleep
Pituitary gland (brain)	Growth hormone	Growth; cell reproduction
Prolactin (brain)	Luteinize hormone	Milk production Sexual gratification
		Stimulates thyroid hormone
		Gland to secrete T3/T4
Thyroid gland (neck)	Thyroxine (T4)	Metabolism: relaxation Range of effects

	Trilodothyronine (T3)	Metabolism: female: ovulation
Adrenal gland (kidney)	Glucocorticoids	Effects glucose uptake
	Adrenaline	Fight-or-flight response (range of effects)
Pancreas (kidney)	Insulin	Regulates glucose
Ovary (female)	Progesterone	Pregnancy, muscle effects
Testes (male)	Testosterone	Muscle mass, bone density
	Androgen	Sexual maturation

When you look at the above chart and see all of the areas affected when the endocrine system is not working properly and with repeated exposure to low- level toxins, you may start with one problem that eventually increases to a compounding of symptoms and problems until you may finally be in a fight for your life. A disruption in your endocrine system can cause conditions and diseases such as diabetes, asthma, rheumatoid arthritis, stroke, and heart attack.

Let's look at an example of toxic overload of the endocrine system. We know that many toxins mimic hormones and can either block the receptor so the hormone cannot deliver the chemical message, or it latches onto the hormone receptor and causes a false response.

Environmental-disrupting chemicals can affect people in many ways: disrupted sexual development, decreased fertility, increased chance of birth defects, reduced immune response, and increased chance of neurological and behavioral changes, including reduced ability to handle stress.

Neurotoxins

Neurotoxins alter neurons, affecting brain activity and causing a range of problems from headaches to loss of intellect. Even minor changes in the structure or function of the nervous system may have profound consequences for neurological, behavioral, and related body functions. Diseases that are examples of neurotoxicity include Parkinson's, Alzheimer's, MS, and ALS.

Symptoms of neurotoxic effects include cognitive effects (memory, learning, and confusion), motor effects (convulsions, weakness, tremor, twitching, lack of coordination, unsteadiness, paralysis, reflex abnormalities, and activity changes), sensory effects (equilibrium changes, vision disorders, pain disorders, tactile disorders, and auditory disorders), mood and personality effects (sleep disturbances, excitability, depression, irritability, restlessness, nervousness, tension, delirium, and hallucinations), and general effects (loss of appetite, depression of neuronal activity, narcosis stupor, fatigue, and nerve damage).

The example of neurotoxicity I am using is me because I spent years going to neurologists, psychologists, internists, family doctors, and seizure specialists trying to find both a cause and a solution to my problem. To illustrate, I will show you two different MRI readings that two different neurologists requested. One was performed in 2004 at St. Luke's Hospital, and the radiologists attributed the scattered white matter appropriate for my age and nonspecific ischemic small vessel ischemic changes plus a large right maxillary sinus mucous retention cyst. I requested these reports years later, but the only thing that was discussed with me was that the brain scan was normal. Nothing would point to any problems.

DATE: 05/21/2004

BRAIN MRI WITHOUT CONTRAST

CLINICAL DATA: Dementia. Question space-occupying lesion.

COMPARISON EXAM: None.

FIELD STRENGTH: 1.5 Tesla

PULSE SEQUENCES: Available on procedure form.

FINDINGS: There are no signs of mass or mass effect. There are no signs of blood or acute/subacute ischemic event. Cortical signal is normal. Note is made of a few scattered areas of punctate white matter signal change approximately 6 and 7 in number within subcortical locations. Brain parenchymal signal is otherwise normal. There appears to be a very mild degree of age-appropriate volume loss. No hydrocephalus. This is a diffuse finding. Vascular flow voids are intact.

No discrete calvarial abnormality identified. Large right maxillary sinus mucous retention cyst noted.

CONCLUSION: 1) Very mild degree of atrophy appropriate for age seen diffusely. A few scattered areas of subcortical white matter signal change are identified. These are nonspecific, but may well represent early chronic small vessel ischemic change. 2) Large right maxillary sinus mucous retention cyst.

IMPRESSION: No acute intracranial pathology. Specifically no intracranial hemorrhage or features of acute cerebral vascular accident. No intracranial mass lesion or midline shift. Tiny focus of nonspecific T2 weighted signal abnormality within the supratentorial brain.

Patient: DIETZLER, JUDITH A
DOB: XX/XX/XXXX
Visit #: XXXXXXX
DOS: XX/XX/XXXX
MR #: XXXXXXXX
Acc. Procedure:

Hosp. Serv.: IDIAVEW
HospitRead: /
P. Date: 7/03/2007 15:00
Exam #: XXXXXXX

Ref. Provider: ROBERT J. DAVIS MD
Add. Provider:
Add. Provider:
Add. Provider:

PROCEDURE: MRI BRAIN W/O AND W CONTRAST

INDICATIONS: Upper extremity and lobectomy numbness and weakness. Slurred speech. Altered mental status.

COMPARISON: Comparison is made with a CT scan of brain performed today.

TECHNIQUE: Precontrast images of the brain were obtained initially, followed by multiphasic gadolinium-enhanced MR imaging with IV administration of 20 cc gadolinium, as detailed in the EHR worksheet.

FINDINGS:

GENERAL COMMENTS:	No evidence of intracranial hemorrhage, acute or chronic cortical infarct, or intracranial mass lesion. No pathologic intracranial enhancement.
VENTRICLES:	Normal in size and morphology.
SUPRATENTORIAL BRAIN:	There is a tiny nonspecific focus of T2 weighted signal abnormality within the left frontal white matter. This is likely the result of chronic microvascular disease.
INFRATENTORIAL BRAIN:	Normal. Cerebellar tonsils are not low lying.
SKULL:	Unremarkable.
MASTOIDS:	Well aerated.
ORBITS:	Normal.
PARANASAL SINUSES:	Well aerated.
ADD'L COMMENTS:	Expected arterial and dural venous sinus flow voids are present.

IMPRESSION: No acute intracranial pathology. Specifically no intracranial hemorrhage or features of acute cerebral vascular accident. No intracranial mass lesion or midline shift. Tiny focus of nonspecific T2 weighted signal abnormality within the supratentorial brain.

In 2007, the MRI was performed at St. Alphonsus Hospital with their conclusion that there was a T2 white matter abnormality within the left frontal lobe as a likely result of chronic microvascular disease.

> **DIAGNOSTIC IMPRESSION:**
>
> Axis I: R/O 290.40 Vascular dementia
> Axis II: V71.09 No diagnosis
> Axis III: None current

My psychologist's report came back as vascular dementia. One of my neurologists sent me to a psychologist two different times over a period of a couple years to test me on different cognitive functions and memory tasks, word games, picture association, and so forth.

I absolutely hated it because, over the years, every time I had symptoms that gave me brain fog for a few hours, it became harder and harder to regain my thought process. I feel that, if I had found the right doctor in 1992 or 1993 or even ten or twelve years ago, recovery from the chemical exposure would have been so much easier.

Instead of having neurotoxicity for twenty-three years, I would have had the same amount of time to heal.

I have to work so much harder now because I have had so many neurological episodes over the years that my brain is in overdrive most of the time.

Neurotoxicity is not uncommon; nor is exposure to mold. However, most people who have it don't realize they have it, so it is just more symptoms that they deal with daily without any answers.

I know how dangerous toxic chemical exposure can be because I deal with the symptoms every single day, but so do you because we are all being exposed daily. The difference is that I am proactive because being passive almost killed me.

If you rely on traditional doctors, the dollar or grocery store, and the pharmaceutical companies, you will have an abundance of toxic chemicals in your system. I have operated my own business since 1975, and for the last twenty-three years, I have a constant daily battle that I am determined to win. I always feel like I have cobwebs and little spiders running through my brain.

Because the mold has affected both my eyes and my brain, I work much harder to compensate in other areas.

Writing this book is a good example. I have a tendency to turn some of my words around and need to reread two or three times before my eyes and brain see the same thing. It really threw me when my editor said I needed to take out all of the pictures and have them in a separate file and just type where the picture is supposed to go, so for two weeks, I had every file open on my desktop, only putting my computer to sleep. I dared not shut it down, or my brain wouldn't remember the sequence of the pages.

So since the book is on the way to the publisher, I am doubling up on all of my detox products, meditating twice a day, going to the chiropractor three times a week, doing BioMat one hour a day, drinking plenty of calming tea, and praying that my mold-infested brain or my editor doesn't allow any keyboard errors to slip from my fingers to your pages.

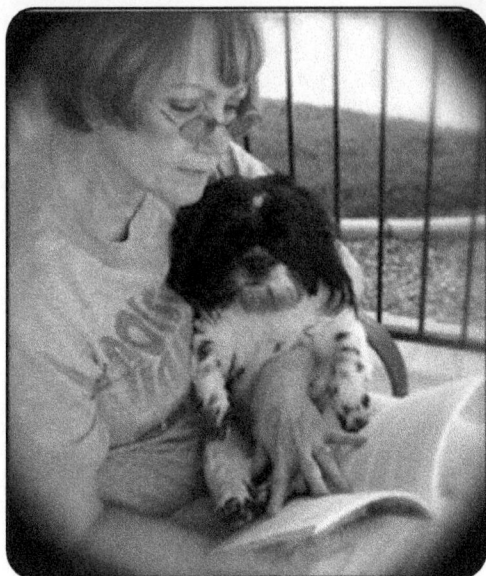

I went to play bingo with friends the other night, and I must tell you that bingo isn't like it used to be. I remember when it was simple, you used pieces of cardboard on the spots, and you shouted "Bingo!" Sounds simple. We got there two hours early so we could draw our diagrams on our bingo cards because they don't play straight bingo. That would be way too easy. They do pretzel, semicolon, bonsai tree, umbrella, and all kinds of weird things I had never heard about, and the bingo caller must have a second job as an auctioneer.

She rattled off those numbers so quickly that I had to hear the number and translate it to the mold-covered brain. The brain had to analyze it (which took a while) and then translate it to the eyes (also covered with mold). The eyes had to quickly scan six cards for the bingo number before her nimble fingers reached for the next ball. By that time, our quick bingo caller had swiftly moved two numbers ahead of me. Did anyone happen to tell the auctioneer bingo caller that this is a senior center filled with seventy-year-olds with arthritis and one of the seniors has mold on the brain?

How much neurotoxicity does your body require and need? None!

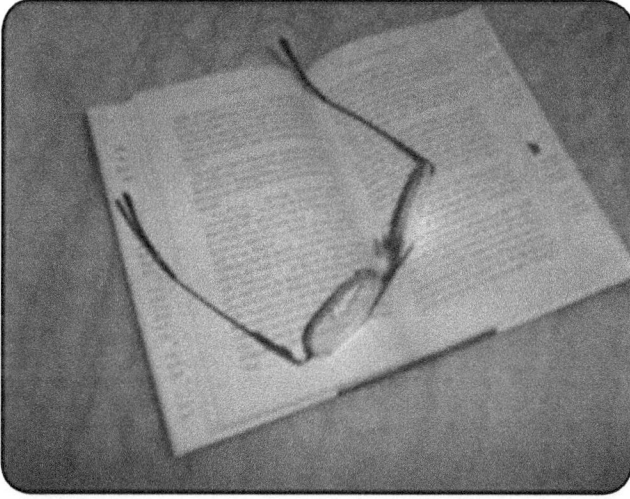

I would like to share the story of a friend I met who is the organizer of a healthy living social meet-up group. She has also been a registered nurse for almost forty years, and like me, Janis has dealt with unexplained health issues for a number of years, including doctor visits, numerous tests, and many unnecessary scans and radiation, leading to disappointment after disappointment. Through her determination and quest for the truth, she started a research journey that she did not plan, but it was a road she needed to travel if she were going to regain her health.

Janis Uquillas, RN

My first toxic exposure was when I was a child picking strawberries in a field in Indiana. I got severe, swollen, thick hives on my face and felt like the inside of my throat and esophagus was burnt. I would pace the floor at night because I felt so miserable with intense itching and burning of my skin. I would put a hot cloth on my face to try to numb the pain. I assumed I was allergic to strawberries, but years later after learning about toxic chemicals, I realized the strawberries are highly sprayed with pesticides. Now I know that I was poisoned with toxic chemicals rather than an allergic reaction because I can eat organic strawberries by the bucket and never have any problem. The chemicals on the strawberries were causing my problems. How many times have we blamed our allergies or illnesses on the wrong thing (for example, strawberries) and deprived ourselves for years when the real problem was toxic chemical exposure?

My next exposure was with cleaning products when our family would clean not only our house but they would also clean other homes in our town. I would be in someone's shower spraying cleaning products, and get dizzy and nauseated. I would start shaking, and then I started having neurological problems at a young age. I would suffer severe attacks of vertigo, which would leave me completely incapacitated. At some point, I developed Lyme disease, but it wasn't diagnosed for almost fifty years. So I went through test after test, doctor after doctor, and diagnosis after diagnosis. I was told I had everything from MS, brain tumor, fibromyalgia, and one mystery diagnosis after another. My symptoms would mimic so many different illnesses, and I couldn't get any answers, but I kept getting sicker as the weeks, months, and years went by.

After I became a nurse and later a medical researcher, I traveled across the country to universities and monitored their studies to make sure they were following FDA regulations. I was reading all of their data, so I've always had an interest in research. For many years, I have been researching toxic chemicals and ingredients.

Even though I was trained in conventional medicine, I have been interested in alternative and holistic medicine. I have always limited what I accept from conventional medicine. I don't like putting any chemicals in or on my body because I was sick for so many years.

I finally started making the connection between chemicals and our environment and what we are putting in our mouth, the products we are using in our homes, our toothpaste, and our personal care products.

I was horrified at what companies are allowed to put in products, even carcinogens and neurotoxins, that I really became passionate on this topic of toxins and how to avoid them. So I try to eat organic, and I started my *own company, JES Organics, because I couldn't find products at the store that met my standards. I didn't set out to start a business or earn a living. My only goal was to have quality products that were chemical and toxin-free, and for me, the only solution was to formulate and manufacture my own. But in the process, I found other people who had the same hopes and desires. I am passionate about educating others about ingredients and toxic chemicals.*

For many years, I have led a large support group for those with chronic illness, and I started seeing more and more the connection between chronic illness and toxic chemical exposure in many others and myself. I continue my research about toxic chemicals and try to educate as many people as possible.

The skin is the largest organ of the body, and consumers need to read the labels, but you also need to be product educated. Marketing sells the product; it doesn't educate you on the product safety. Watch what you put on your skin and in your mouth. And watch what you use in your home. If you can't buy organic products, you need to at least wash and scrub your products with a natural, nontoxic, chemical-free spray to remove the chemicals. And whatever you do, don't use cleaning products that have toxic chemicals in them that you will inhale or absorb into your skin. You could also flush them down the drain, which will hurt our environment and wildlife.

The government says that the chemical exposure in our food and household products is at acceptable limits, but what they don't seem to understand is that your body is accumulating multiple toxins, so if you have one product with a toxin in it, according to the government, that is an acceptable limit. But if you take that times twenty more products, how does that affect your acceptable limit? It's an accumulative affect, and I believe that chronic illness is due to the accumulative effect of all of the toxins we are exposed to daily. Studies have tested the fetal-cord blood of newborn babies, and babies are being born already contaminated with numerous toxic chemicals. It's huge, and the manufacturers and the government are underplaying it.

For readers who are not familiar with Lyme disease, Lyme disease is a bacterial infection that is transmitted through the bite of a tick. Lyme disease is best treated in the early stages, but in Janis's case, it wasn't even diagnosed for nearly fifty years. Early symptoms are chills, fever, enlarged lymph nodes, sore throat, vision changes, fatigue, muscle, aches, and headaches. As the disease progresses, there are also additional symptoms like arthritis, disturbances in the heart rhythm, brain disorders involving memory, mood and sleep, short-term memory loss, difficulty concentrating, mental fogginess, problems following conversation, and numbness in the arms, legs, hands, or feet. Lyme disease can attack literally every bodily function.

There is a pattern. When Janis goes to the doctor, she is worked up for and sometimes diagnosed with illnesses that mimic well-known diseases. They have similar characteristics, but they are also dissimilar. She has tests and blood work to confirm the diagnosis, but the results come back normal, which makes no sense if you are the patient and you are sick and can barely function. But the doctor is telling you that he or she can't find anything wrong with you. Janis used to tell the doctors, "I look great on paper, but I feel like crap."

So the only conclusion the doctor can come to is that you are depressed or anxious or need antidepressants or sleeping pills. So out the door you go with your new friend (more chemicals), but you still have a toxic overload that hasn't come close to being diagnosed or addressed.

Lessons I've Learned in My Life!

Life may not always bring you sunshine and rainbows, but if you wait out the storm long enough, they always appear if you look for them.

Chapter 5 Review

1. Does the Environmental Protection Agency regulate household chemicals and test them for safety? What are the three internal factors that cause cancer?

   _____

   _____

2. What are the four external factors that cause cancer?

   _____

   _____

3. Toxic chemicals can mimic hormones, confusing the body with false signals that are called endocrine disruptors. Endocrine disruptors can lead to numerous health concerns, including:

   _____

   _____

4. A disruption in your endocrine system can cause conditions and diseases such as:

   a.) Diabetes b.) Asthma c.) Rheumatoid arthritis d.) Stroke e.) Heart attack f.) All of the above

   _____

   _____

5. Which of the following are either diseases or symptoms of neurotoxicity?
   a) Parkinson's   b) Alzheimer's
   c) Convulsions   d) Multiple sclerosis
   e) Vision disorders   f) Nerve damage
   g) Pain disorders   h) Depression
   i) Fatigue   j) Sleep disturbance
   k) Confusion   l) Unsteadiness
   m) Amyotrophic sclerosis (ALS)   n) All of the above

6

WHERE ARE THE TOXIC CHEMICALS IN YOUR HOME?

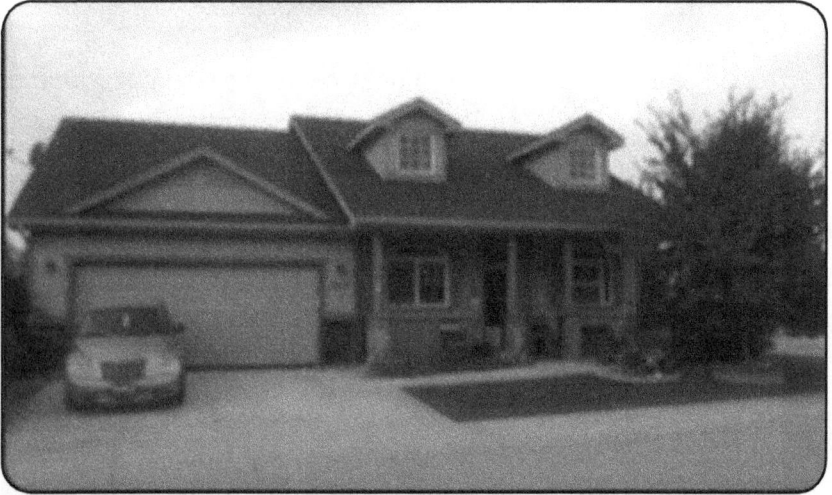

When you look at your house, I am sure it looks safe and secure. I am sure you feel safe when you go home.

The first room you come to in my house is my kitchen, and it looks harmless enough, but until I removed all of the toxic chemicals from my home, my kitchen was the most dangerous room in the house. I always sprayed 409 cleaner on the counters, stove, and cabinets. I sprayed Comet on the sink and used Cascade automatic dishwashing detergent, Pine Sol, and so forth. Every product said, "Keep out of reach of children." So the house looked safe, but it was anything but safe for my family and my pets.

Bisphenol A (BPA)

This is a chemical used in plastic production, and it is found in water bottles, baby bottles, plastic wraps, and food packaging. The government's national toxicology program has concluded that there is some concern about brain and behavioral effects on fetuses and young children at current exposure levels. As a better alternative, switch to glass products when possible.

Ammonia

A very volatile chemical, ammonia is very damaging to your eyes, respiratory tract, and skin.

All-Purpose Cleaner

Health effects include irritation and/or damage to the skin, eyes, and lungs. The fumes can cause dizziness and feelings of light-headedness, and chronic irritation may occur from repeated use. Some all-purpose cleaners contain the sudsing agents diethanolamine (DEA) and triethanolamine (TEA), which can react with nitrites (an often undisclosed preservative or contaminant) to form nitrosamines carcinogens that readily penetrate the skin. Skin also easily absorbs nerve-damaging butyl cellosolve (also known as ethylene glycol monobutyl ether), present in some cleaners. Fumes from ammonia-containing cleaners may cause respiratory irritation. Sodium hydroxide and sodium hypochlorite (bleach) are highly caustic, and sodium hypochlorite should never be mixed with any product containing ammonia or acids, or toxic gases will result. To prevent chemical accidents, it's best to simply avoid.

These detergents, disinfectants, and solvents often contain the following hazardous ingredients: ammonia, ethylene glycol monobutyl acetate, sodium hypochlorite, 2-butoxy ethanol, and trisodium phosphate.

Most household cleaning needs can be met safely and inexpensively with a sturdy scrubber sponge and simple ingredients like water, vinegar, lemon juice, or baking soda for scrubbing grease and grime.

Automatic Dishwashing Detergents

If swallowed, these detergents can cause mild to severe internal burns and are harmful to the environment. Most mainstream dishwashing detergents are petroleum-based, contributing to the depletion of this nonrenewable resource and our nation's dependence on imported oil.

The detergents may contain bleach, sodium carbonate, and heavy fragrances, which can cause irritation to skin and the lungs over time. The detergents are also alkaline, which may classify them as corrosive toxins. They also contain phosphates and are known to harm the environment.

Look for plant-based detergents instead. Opt for colorless liquids. Dyes can be contaminated with heavy metals such as arsenic and lead and may penetrate the skin during washing and leave impurities on dishes.

Powdered detergents for automatic dishwashers can contain phosphates, which overnutrify rivers and streams, causing excessive algae growth that deprives fish of oxygen. Those made with chlorine can release steamy chlorinated chemicals into the air when the dishwasher is opened at the end of the wash cycle.

Floor Cleaner

Floor cleaner can irritate skin, eyes, throat mucous membranes, and the respiratory tract. Inhalation causes headache and drowsiness.

Toxic ingredients may include pine oil, petroleum distillates, naphtha, and irritants to the eyes, skin, throat, mucous membranes, and respiratory tract. Inhalation and prolonged use may cause drowsiness, headaches, pulmonary edema, and, in extreme cases, coma or cardiac arrest.

Isopropyl Alcohol

Isopropyl alcohol, or isopropanol, is highly flammable and found in many cleaning agents plus some rubbing alcohols. With absorption through the skin, prolonged inhalation, or oral ingestion in large quantities, it may produce symptoms such as headaches, dizziness, mental depression, nausea, vomiting, and, in extreme cases, coma.

Oven Cleaner

The fumes and vapors are extremely toxic and irritating to the skin, eyes, and lungs. Contact with the skin can cause moderate to serious burns. Inhalation causes irritation to the nose, mouth, and lungs, causing headache, coughing, nausea, and vomiting. Ingestion is fatal.

Prevent spills from being baked onto the oven floor by lining it with aluminum foil and cleaning them up before they have had time to dry and cook. To remove grease and charred food residues without resorting to caustic chemicals, try soaking oven surfaces overnight in a mixture of water, baking soda, and soap and then scrubbing off with baking soda and a soapy sponge. Or a paste of washing soda and water may do the trick, but be sure to wear gloves when working with washing soda.

It contains sodium hydroxide (forms of lye) and/or potassium hydroxide, which are extremely caustic and corrosive. Contact with the skin or eyes causes burning sensations. Inhalation causes burning and irritation to nose and lungs, and it has long-term effects on vital internal organs.

Scouring Powder

Inhaling the fumes may be highly irritating to the eyes, skin, and respiratory tract. It can be fatal if mixed with ammonia. Some scouring powders contain silica, which is harmful when inhaled, as the abrasive scrubbing agent. And some are made with chlorine bleach, which may irritate skin and airways and will form hazardous gases if mixed with ammonia or acidic cleaners.

Scouring powder may contain calcium carbonate and chlorine bleach. Fumes from these chemicals can be extremely irritating to the eyes and respiratory tract. It can cause irritation and redness to the skin. Any combination with products containing ammonia (such as toilet bowl cleaner or all-purpose cleaners) produces chloramine gas, which can be fatal.

Toxic organic solvents common to household products include benzene, toluene, xylene, isopropyl alcohol, methanol, chlorinated hydrocarbons, naphtha, petroleum solvents, turpentine, and acetone. Over time, health effects may include liver and kidney problems, birth defects, nervous disorders, central nervous system damage, and, in severe cases, unconsciousness and death.

Solvents are extremely hazardous. Vapors are easily inhaled and may cause irritation to the eyes, nose, mouth, and lungs. Many solvents have toxic constituents that have long-term effects on the liver and kidneys.

Baking soda effectively scours away most grime on tubs, showers, toilets, and countertops. For cleaning up grease, cleaning expert Annie Berthold-Bond recommends applying a mixture of a half teaspoon of washing soda, two tablespoons of distilled white vinegar, one-quarter teaspoon liquid soap, and two cups of hot water with a spray bottle. Wear gloves when working with washing soda though. Or try the following brands. Bon Ami can be found in grocery others at natural foods stores.

Oxybenzone

This is a chemical used in cosmetics and found in sunscreens, lip balm, and moisturizers. It is linked to hormone disruption and low–birth weight babies. About 97 percent of Americans have the compound in their urine, but current exposure levels have been deemed safe. But that could change.

Fluoride

Fluoride is a form of the basic element fluorine and is found in toothpaste and tap water. It is neurotoxic and potentially tumorigenic if swallowed.

The American Dental Association advises that children under two not use fluoride toothpaste.

Government studies support current fluoride levels in tap water, but studies on long-term exposure and cancers are ongoing.

Butylated Hydroxyanisole (BHA)

BHA is an additive that preserves fats and oils in food and cosmetics, and it is found in chewing gum, snack foods, and diaper creams. It may promote cancer in lab animals. BHA is hard to avoid in foods, but the government limits its levels.

Parabens

They are synthetic preservatives found in products like moisturizers and hair care and shaving products. It causes hormone disruptions and cancer in animals. The FDA has deemed current levels in cosmetics safe, but paraben-free products are available.

Antibacterial Cleaners

These cleaners may contain triclosan, and absorption through the skin can be tied to liver damage.

Drain Cleaner

Chemical drain cleaners are among the most dangerous of all cleaning products. Most contain corrosive ingredients such as sodium hydroxide and sodium hypochlorite (bleach) that can permanently burn eyes and skin. Some can be fatal if ingested.

Prevent drains from becoming blocked in the first place by capturing hair and other drain-clogging particles with inexpensive metal or plastic drain screens, available at home improvement and hardware stores. Regularly collect and dispose of hair that collects around shower or sink drains, and do not allow large food scraps to wash down the kitchen sink.

When clogs occur, use a snake plumbing tool to manually remove blockage, or try suction removal with a plunger. If you purchase a chemical drain cleaner, choose one of the two below that use enzymes, rather than caustic chemicals, to eat away gunk. Earth Friendly is available in natural foods stores; Naturally Yours must be ordered by mail. Like chemical cleaners, these are most effective on drains that are only partly clogged.

Drain cleaners often contain caustic ingredients including lye, hydrochloric acid, trichloroethane, and sulfuric acid. Fumes can cause prolonged irritation to the eyes, nose, and lungs, and if ingested, it will damage the esophagus and stomach. Avoid contact with the skin and eyes as the corrosive chemicals can cause burns, nausea, and blindness in addition to damaging the liver and kidneys.

Hair Spray

Hair spray can be highly flammable. Health effects from long-term use may include irritation to eyes and respiratory system as well as serious health problems. It may contain harmful aerosols and polyvinylpyrrolidone, which has been associated with brain, kidney, and liver damage.

Nail Polish Remover

Nail polish remover is flammable and irritating to eyes, nose, and throat. It contains acetone and ethyl acetate. Both ingredients are flammable and highly toxic if ingested. Continued use causes lung irritation, anesthetic effects, and brittle nails.

Toilet Bowl Cleaner

Toilet bowl cleaner can include hydrochloric acid or sodium acid sulfate, and it is extremely toxic and corrosive. These chemicals can burn the skin and cause blindness if splashed in the eyes or can burn the stomach if ingested. If it is inhaled, it can be a strong irritant to the eyes and respiratory tract. Some toilet bowl cleaners contain sulfates, which may trigger asthma attacks in those with asthma. Toxic ingredients include sodium bisulfate, oxalic acid 5%, 5- dimethyldantoin, hydrochloric acid, and phenol. These chemicals and their fumes are extremely toxic, carcinogenic, and corrosive. Long-term effects include damage to the kidney and liver, respiratory tract irritation, central nervous system depression, and severe circulatory system damage. It is corrosive to the mouth, skin, mucous membranes, and stomach.

I hear a lot of people say that they can't possibly be getting exposed to very many toxins, but let's take a look at it and see if we can narrow it down a bit. I counted how many products I used in the morning just to get ready to face the world. Before I left the bathroom, I used twenty-seven items. In your case, that would be twenty-seven items with toxic chemicals.

You still have several rooms to walk through and so many more toxins before your day has even started. Once you add cleaning products to the mix, the toxins will keep accumulating until your body reaches the breaking point.

Air Fresheners

Health effects from exposure to air fresheners include irritation to the eyes, throat, and lungs. Fumes act as a nerve-deadening agent to cover up one smell with another, but they can be very damaging to the respiratory tract. It is highly toxic, a known carcinogen. It is reported to also have phenol. When phenol touches your skin, it can cause it to swell, burn, peel, and break out in hives, and it can cause cold sweats, convulsions, circulatory collapse, coma, and even death.

Aerosol sprays are easily inhaled and absorbed into the body and usually are flammable. Fragrances can provoke asthmatic or allergic reactions in sensitive individuals.

To clear out odors, improve ventilation by opening windows and using fans. Baking soda is good at removing odors, and spritzes of lemon or any citrus fruit freshens air. Wooden cedar blocks, pure essential oils, or sachets of natural dried flowers or herbs (such as aromatic roses, lavender, and lemon verbena) provide gentler fragrance. Read labels.

Air fresheners often contain the carcinogenic toxin formaldehyde, which strongly irritates the eyes, throat, skin, and lungs. Other ingredients may include petroleum distillates, P-dichlorobenzene, and aerosol propellants, all of which act as respiratory irritants and may cause lung and/ or liver damage and even brain damage if inhaled in high concentrations or for prolonged periods of time.

Bleach

Contact with eyes can cause severe irritation and burns. Fumes can be a strong irritant to eyes, throat, and lungs. Ingestion can cause injury to the esophagus and stomach, resulting in nausea and vomiting. It contains chlorine, which can cause irritation to the eyes, nose, and respiratory system. Bleach mixed with acidic substances found in other cleaners creates toxic fumes, leading to coughing, burning sensations in the throat and lungs, suffocation, and, in severe cases, death.

Laundry Detergent

Laundry detergent can be an irritant to the skin. If swallowed, it can cause mild to severe internal burning, and it is harmful to the environment. It may contain enzymes and heavy fragrances, which can cause sensitization or irritation to skin and, over time, to the lungs. Industrial exposure can cause dermatitis and asthma. It also contains phosphates, which are harmful to the environment.

They say you can't remove stains unless you use toxic products because nothing else is effective, but that isn't true. That is what the advertisers would like you to believe. For example, lemon juice can remove rust. Applying diluted juice or orange water can remove grease and oil. For food stains, quickly grab some soda water and apply it over the stain. For ink, you need to dab on rubbing alcohol. In the case of wax, let it cool first and then remove each layer one by one using an iron and a newspaper. In the case of tarnish, a paste of baking soda or toothpaste is used to brush on.

Spot Remover

Fumes are acutely toxic and carcinogenic. Symptoms of inhalation may include dizziness, sleepiness, nausea, loss of appetite, and disorientation. Hazardous ingredients may include perchloroethylene, which emits carcinogenic and toxic fumes. Prolonged or chronic use can result in liver damage or central nervous system depression. Exposure to the skin can result in redness and chapping.

Furniture Polish

Skin contact with furniture polishes can cause irritation, and many brands contain nerve-damaging petroleum distillates, which are flammable and dangerous if swallowed. Some formulations may contain formaldehyde, a suspected carcinogen. Aerosol spray furniture polishes are easily inhaled into lung tissue.

Depending on whether polish is a solvent, emulsion, or aerosol, it may contain several of the following toxic ingredients: ammonia, naphtha, nitrobenzene, petroleum distillates, and phenol. Long-term inhalation and/or contact with the skin may include chronic irritation to the respiratory tract, liver damage, and even skin and lung cancer.

For dusting and polishing, combine a mix of a half cup white vinegar and one teaspoon olive oil (or less if this ratio leaves your wood furniture too oily). Or look for solvent-free products that use plant oils as the active polish. Look for Earth Friendly at natural foods stores, or order by mail.

Furniture Cleaner

Furniture cleaner contains flammable propellants, and it is an irritant to the skin, eyes, and respiratory tract. Hazardous ingredients include petroleum distillates and oil of cedar, which irritates the skin, eyes, and lungs and may cause fatal pulmonary edema. It may induce spontaneous abortion in pregnant women and acts as a central nervous system depressant.

Glass Window Cleaner

The fumes from window cleaner can cause irritation to the skin, eyes, and lungs. Some window cleaners contain nerve-damaging butyl cellosolve. Many contain ammonia, which may irritate airways and will release toxic chloramine gases if accidentally mixed with chlorine-containing cleaners.

Most window cleaners contain ammonia and isopropanol alcohol, which can irritate the eyes, lungs, and the body's mucous membranes and can cause rashes or burns on the skin after prolonged use. Ingestion may result in drowsiness, nausea, unconsciousness, and even death.

Plain water is just as effective as some commercial glass cleaners. Or fill your own spray bottle with water and either one-quarter cup white vinegar or one tablespoon of lemon juice to help wipe away greasy fingerprints and other harder- to-remove spots.

Insect Repellent

Insect repellant is an irritant to sensitive skin and toxic to the respiratory tract. Ingestion or inhalation can cause central nervous system depression and may affect the liver and kidneys. Excessive use can produce symptoms such as loss of coordination, anxiety, behavioral changes, and mental confusion. Active ingredients include butopyronoxyl, cimethyl phthalate, and diethyltoluamide (DEET). Long-term effects from these toxins can cause mild necrosis in the liver and kidney. Ingestion of large doses or prolonged use may cause loss of coordination, central nervous system depression, and possibly coma.

Insecticide

Insecticide is an extremely toxic carcinogen. Symptoms of inhalation include dizziness, headache, twitching, and nausea. Ingredients in insecticides may include organophosphates and carbamates. These are acutely toxic and carcinogenic. Long-term health effects include damage to the nervous system, headache, nausea, and lung irritation.

Mildew Remover

This is a strong corrosive toxin and suspected carcinogen. Health effects from inhalation, absorption through the skin, or ingestion can cause respiratory irritation, including lung inflammation, and dry skin. Ingredients may include phenol, kerosene, sodium hypochlorite, formaldehyde, and pentachlorophenol, which are extremely toxic, causing long-term health challenges such as central nervous system depression, lung inflammation, and circulatory system problems. Phenol is corrosive to the skin and a suspected carcinogen; pentachlorophenol is toxic to unborn children, even causing birth defects.

Roach Killer

This is an acutely toxic pesticide suspected to be carcinogenic. Inhalation can cause headaches, dizziness, nausea, and/ or twitching, and it affects the nervous system. It contains organophosphates and carbonates, both of which are suspected carcinogens and mutagenic. Reports have also found teratogenicity in dogs and chick embryos.

Rodent Killer

This toxin, which contains warfarin, is both hazardous to our environment and fish and, if ingested in large amounts, causes internal bleeding.

I was going to a meeting with one of my friends, and we were talking about toxins and the effect they can have on the body. I mentioned the fact that not everyone will have the severity of symptoms that I have, but everyone has toxic chemicals in his or her body that is causing damage. She immediately said that, in order for the body to suffer any kind of damage, you would need to ingest a large dose all at one time. Her response isn't uncommon. You can get exposed to a chemical in a devastating single dose maybe through a national disaster, but that isn't the only time you are going to be exposed to toxins. Most people probably don't realize that when you accumulate small doses of toxic substances—including chemicals, toxins, junk food and negativity from toxic people—over decades, your body will respond negatively with one symptom after another until you either pay attention and change your response or habits or until your body eventually shuts down.

Read Labels: If you can't pronounce it, you probably shouldn't use it!

Tips to Help Eliminate Toxic Chemicals in Your Home

It's simple to stay away from something harmful when you can see it with your own eyes; however, what about the things you can't see, like the toxic substances lurking in everything we purchase on a regular basis? As we go about our daily routine, toxic products that compromise our health and the health of our family constantly bombard us. It is our responsibility to protect our family from harsh and toxic chemicals. Ultimately, it is not the government's job to keep the toxins from walking through our front door and becoming a resident in our home.

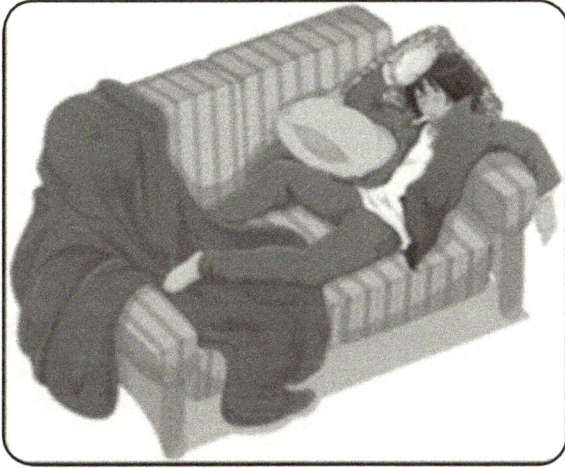

The following easy methods help you limit chemical exposure. Adopt these simple ideas to create a cleaner, safer world for you and your family.

Kitchen

- **Purchase BPA-free.** When buying plastic baby bottles, sippy cups, water bottles, or food storage containers, make certain they say BPA-free on the label. Better yet, search for glass or stainless steel.

- **Toss your Teflon in the trash.** Most nonstick cookware is made utilizing PFOAs (perfluorooctanoic acid), a toxic chemical linked to most cancers causing many different health issues. Select stainless steel or enameled pots and pans instead.

- **Don't microwave plastic.** Heat causes chemical substances to leach out of plastic containers and into food. Be on the safe side and keep away from plastic in the microwave completely.

Inside Your House

- **Remove your shoes.** Take your footwear off at the door to keep pesticides and other chemicals from spreading toxins throughout your home.

- **Change to toxic-free cleaning products.** I purchase all of my cleaning, body and hair care, and nutritional products from a manufacturer that makes only toxic- free products. They are out there, but most don't advertise. Search for products made with plant-based ingredients.

- **Dust, vacuum, and mop regularly.** Whereas these might not be your favorite activities, they do cut down on toxic substances that can accumulate in your home.

- **Take care with upholstery.** Most upholstery comprises flame-retardant chemical compounds, and many are toxic. Reduce exposure by getting rid of old, outdated furniture with flame-retardant chemicals. Instead, you may want to choose wool, jute, or cotton as your upholstery choice because they are natural flame-retardants.

- **Skip the stain protectors.** Stain-resistant chemical substances used on and in fabrics include toxic PFOAs that accumulate in household dust.

- **Keep away from volatile compounds (VOCs).** They're the one thing you shouldn't breathe. VOCs are present in paints, air fresheners, and numerous other products. They're typically used in dry cleaning processes.

Our Children

- **Keep away from phthalates.** When buying toys for your little one, avoid the words *vinyl* and *PVC*. They are used to soften the plastic, and they are toxic. That plasticky odor is another dead giveaway.

- **Choose wood carefully.** Wood toys are classic and wonderful, but when they're treated with petrochemical sealants, they may be toxic for children to chew on. Search for wooden handles with nontoxic finishes like beeswax or linseed oil instead. Select solid wood over manufactured wood that may release toxic formaldehyde fumes.

- Purchase nontoxic craft supplies. Say no to oil- based paints that give off harmful fumes and polymer clay made with phthalates. Say yes to water- based play paints, natural fabric material cloth dyes, and homemade play dough.

I remember my determination to finally solve my mystery symptoms when I flew to Mayo Clinic in October 2010. They spent hours asking me a series of questions and finally admitted me to a floor for observation. But I was utterly dismayed and surprised when I found that I was on the seizure ward hooked up to tons of electrodes, because I had spent a week in an Idaho hospital two years earlier. Seizures were ruled out, so they were wasting their time, but they kept electrodes attached to my head. Finally six days into this adventure, I told them that if they wanted to see me have an episode all they needed to do was give me Tegretol, a seizure medication. For some reason, it would cause me to have the symptoms that I was trying to avoid.

One of my neurologists had prescribed Tegretol a few years earlier, and my symptoms increased to the point where I couldn't get out of bed without having them. My doctor didn't figure out that the problem was the medicine. I discovered that the symptoms were worse soon after I took the medicine, and later in the day, the symptoms lessened. When I stopped taking the medicine, the symptoms stopped.

So the attending doctor gave me Tegretol on Saturday, and by Sunday, I was having symptoms. Soon they decided that I was not having seizures. That was what I told them a week earlier when I arrived at the hospital, so on Monday morning, they released me to go home without a diagnosis.

I now had a really big concern. I was in Phoenix by myself, and I fly standby, which means I go out to the airport and hope I can get on a flight. I told them I was concerned that the Tegretol might still be in my system and could cause me to have symptoms, but they assured me that would not be a problem because the Tegretol was no longer in my system.

I was wheeled down to the waiting shuttle, and off to the airport I went. I no sooner got to the airport than I realized I couldn't walk. The shuttle driver needed to get me a wheelchair. He found someone to escort me to the gate where I waited until my flight was getting ready to board. Then I had another dilemma that I needed to overcome. I had to figure out how to get on the plane because I still couldn't walk or talk very well. A nice little lady with silver gray hair was sitting next to me.

I leaned over to her and asked, "Ma'am, could I ask a favor?" She promptly smiled and said, "Yes."

I told her, "I have a neurological problem, and at the moment, I can't walk or talk very well. I really need to get on that plane, but I fly standby. Could you take my ticket to them and let them know I was here? Could you tell them I would also need someone to help me get on the plane?"

She grabbed my ticket, and off she went to solve my most immediate problem. She was certainly sent from heaven. Without her, I would probably still be sitting in the Phoenix airport. She jumped into action, rushed to the podium, handed the gate agent my ticket, and made sure they handed her my boarding pass. She then rushed over and grabbed a sturdy wheelchair attendant, told him she had an emergency, and gave me a hug, and off to my flight I was whisked and placed gently in row one headed for Denver.

Next stop was the Denver airport, and as we landed, I was thrilled that I was closer to home. But I still couldn't walk, so I told the flight attendant I would need a wheelchair with a female driver because she would need to help maneuver me through the bathroom maze. I was then parked at my next location, the flight that would take me to my home state of Idaho.

When I have neurological symptoms, they usually last for three or four hours, and then I'm back to what most people would consider normal, but it had been well over four hours with no signs that my symptoms planned to let up anytime in the near future. When the next flight was called, I was close enough to the customer service agent that he pushed my wheelchair on the plane bound for Boise. It wasn't until that moment that I actually sighed in relief and knew I would make it home.

Lessons I've Learned in My Life!

You can't be both a friend and a gossip! Friendship builds relationships; gossip kills them.

Chapter 6 Review

1. Name four products in your kitchen that have toxic chemicals in them or warning labels on them.

   _____

   _____

   _____

   _____

2. Name four products in your laundry/bathroom that have toxic chemicals in them or warning labels on them.

   _____

   _____

   _____

   _____

3. What are seven of the twelve tips to eliminate toxic chemicals from your home?

   1._____   2._____

   3._____   4._____

   5._____   6._____

   7._____

7

KNOWLEDGE IS POWER

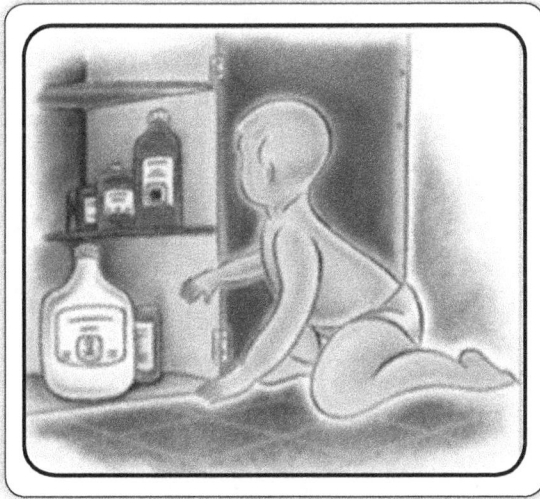

"Life is change. Growth is optional. Choose wisely."

Read labels. According to Dr. Ben Kim, the following are among the most common household toxins (http:// drbenkim.com/ articles-household-toxins.htm):

- **Pesticides.** According to the Environmental Protection Agency (EPA), 60 percent of herbicides, 90 percent of fungicides, and 30 percent of insecticides are known to be carcinogenic. Alarmingly, pesticide residues have been detected in 50–95 percent of US foods. They can cause cancer, developmental challenges, and reproductive problems.

- **Mold and Other Fungal Toxins.** 33 percent of people have had an allergic reaction to mold. Mycotoxins (fungal toxins) can cause a range of health problems with exposure to only a small amount. It can cause cancer, heart disease, asthma, multiple sclerosis, and diabetes. Major sources include contaminated buildings, food like peanuts, wheat, corn and alcoholic beverages, and saline breast implants.

- **Phthalates.** Large phthalates are chemicals that are added to plastics to impart resilience and flexibility. Smaller phthalates prolong the length of time that a scented product maintains fragrance. They have been linked to endocrine, reproductive, and developmental problems. They are endocrine disruptors and carcinogenic and most commonly found in vinyl flooring; plastic food packaging, bags, and clothing; detergents, children's toys, shower curtains, and personal care products like soap, shampoo, nail polish, and hair spray.

- **Volatile Organic Compounds (VOCs).** VOCs are chemicals that are released into the air as gases. They are linked to reproductive, respiratory, neurological, and developmental problems. They are also linked to different types of cancer. They are most commonly found in air fresheners, hairspray, perfumes, cleaning products, paints, carpets, and furniture made out of pressed wood. They can cause cancer, eye and respiratory tract irritation, headaches, dizziness, visual disorders, and memory impairment. Major sources are drinking water, carpet, paints, deodorants, cleaning fluids, varnishes, cosmetics, perfumes, air fresheners, disinfectants, deodorizers, dry-cleaned clothing, moth repellants, and air fresheners.

- **Heavy Metals.** Metals like arsenic, mercury, lead, aluminum, and cadmium, which are prevalent in many areas of our environment, can accumulate in soft tissues of the body. They may cause cancer, neurological disorders, Alzheimer's, foggy head, fatigue, nausea and vomiting, decreased production of red and white blood cells, abnormal heart rhythm, and blood vessel damage. Major sources are drinking water, fish, vaccines, pesticides, preserved wood, antiperspirant, building materials, and dental amalgams.

- **Formaldehyde.** Formaldehyde is commonly known as a preservative. Many people do not know that it is also a germicide, bactericide, and fungicide, among other functions. Formaldehyde is found in household cleaners and disinfectants. It is also present in nail polish and other personal care products. Formaldehyde is a carcinogen.

- **Phenol and Cresol.** These are found in disinfectants, and if ingested, they can cause diarrhea, fainting, dizziness, and kidney and liver damage. When phenol touches your skin, it can cause swelling and burning in addition to peeling and breaking out in hives. It can also cause cold sweats, convulsions, circulatory collapse, coma, and even death. They may cause sore throat, coughing, eye and skin irritation, rapid breathing, bronchi narrowing, wheezing, blue coloring of the skin, accumulation of fluid in the lungs, pain in the lung region, severe eye and skin burns, lung collapse, and reactive airways dysfunction syndrome (RADS) (a type of asthma). Major sources are household cleaners, drinking water (in small amounts), and air when living near an industry (such as a paper plant) that uses chlorine in industrial processes.

- **Carbon Monoxide**. This is formed from incomplete combustion of fuel. Carbon monoxide decreases delivery of oxygen to cells. It is linked to cardiovascular and nervous system failure. It is most commonly produced by leaking furnaces and chimneys, gas stoves, wood stoves and fireplaces, back-drafting from gas water heaters, and auto exhaust from an attached garage or nearby traffic.

- **Bisphenol A.** This is used in epoxy resins that line some metal cans and is used to make polycarbonate plastics utilized in a variety of food containers and baby products. It is linked to endocrine problems. It is most commonly found in food and drink containers, baby bottles, toys, metal food cans, and dental sealants used to prevent cavities.

- **Perfluorinated Chemicals.** They are used to make stain repellents and nonstick surfaces. They are linked to many different types of cancer and developmental problems in children. They are most commonly found in Teflon-coated cookware, microwave popcorn bags, and stain-guarded clothing, furniture, and carpets. Symptoms of toxicity include headache, backache, stiff joints, nausea, diarrhea, asthma, allergies, dizziness, memory loss, stuttering, premature puberty, dyslexia, low sperm count, autism, ADHD, birth defects, antisocial behavior, and sudden mood swings.

Carcinogenic Chemicals (Cancer- Causing Chemicals)

Hundreds of chemicals, even thousands of them, are capable of causing cancer to occur in test animals and humans alike. Cancer seldom eventuates from one acute exposure, but after prolonged low-level exposure or exposure over shorter periods at higher levels. There are many well-known and documented examples of chemicals that actually cause cancer in humans. For example, the fumes of the metals cadmium, nickel, and chromium will cause lung cancer. Vinyl chloride can cause sarcomas, while the exposure to arsenic substantially increases the risk of skin and lung cancer.

Chemically induced changes in bone marrow by toxic chemicals such as benzene and cyclophosphamide and other toxic chemicals result in leukemia. Scientific organizations funded by governments consider benzo[a]pyrene and ethylene dibromide to be carcinogenic to humans as they are potent carcinogens in test animals.

The sad fact of the matter is that cancer induced by chemicals takes many years to establish and may not become apparent until long after the chronic low-level exposure has stopped, as may be the case with an infant crawling on surfaces that have been cleaned with toxic chemicals used by an unaware mother.

A good example of the latency period involved with one particularly bad carcinogen is the length of time it takes for lung cancer to develop after acute or chronic exposure to asbestos or to the more well-known example of cigarette smoke. A latency period of as much as thirty years is common for many of today's known carcinogens.

It took at least thirty-five years before the FDA decided that cigarette smoking was harmful to your health, and every time smoke was inhaled, carcinogenic chemicals were filling your body. It will take longer than thirty-five years before you will see warning labels on the doors of plastic surgeons' offices stating breast implants are proven to be endocrine disruptors, cause neurotoxicity, and can cause cancer. "Purchase at your own risk." This is a woman's issue, so don't expect Congress and the FDA to work very fast on it.

I could write a book on all of the women who are sick because they were sold a dream and ended up with a nightmare. The saddest part of the story is that, when they asked for help, instead of trying to help their patients get better, the doctors told them it must be stress or anxiety and gave them toxic antidepressants and sent them home. Not one doctor said, "Let's run some tests and see if there is a chance that the problem could be caused due to your breast implants. Maybe we should consider a toxicology panel to see if you are sensitive to the silicone shells, or if there's a chance of mold due to saline leakage." It all starts with asking the right questions.

Over the years, I spent a fair amount of money on doctors trying to find the answers to my health questions, and in the process, I did come up with a couple of important insights:

- If my doctor doesn't have a great bedside manner, then he or she doesn't deserve my money.

- If my doctor doesn't have the time to answer my questions, then he or she doesn't deserve my money.

- If the staff at my doctor's office doesn't give good service, then my doctor doesn't deserve my money.

I made an amazing discovery while researching the material for this book. I knew how I became ill and the path it took, and finally it was determined that basilar migraines were causing me to have TIAs (mini strokes) that lasted three to four hours.

But when I found the information on how toxins alter neurons, affecting brain activity and causing a range of problems from headaches to loss of memory and stroke-like symptoms, I was literally stopped in my tracks. I found a symptomatic match.

Symptoms of neurotoxic effects include *loss of memory, learning problems, confusion*, convulsions, *weakness*, tremor, *twitching, lack of coordination, unsteadiness*, paralysis, reflex abnormalities, activity changes, *equilibrium changes, vision disorders, pain disorders*, tactile disorders, auditory disorders, *sleep disturbances*, excitability, depression, irritability, *restlessness*, nervousness, tension, delirium, hallucinations, loss of appetite, depression of neuronal activity, narcosis stupor, *fatigue, and nerve damage.*

At least half of the symptoms that are listed under neurotoxins are the exact symptoms that I have (italics), so even though my symptoms mimic TIAs, they actually indicated neurotoxicity. The symptoms also increased over time. I studied and passed my insurance and securities licensing exams. I was licensed to be a financial advisor the first time I took the exam, and many people retook the exam two or three times before they passed. But every time I have had a neurological episode, it has taken a little more of my memory, and it gets a little harder for me to bounce back.

Earlier in the book, I said I always took the reports showing the psychological tests, EEGs, and MRIs all highlighted because I felt they held the key to finding the solution to my problem. In May 2013, while working on the final draft of my book, I traveled to Atlanta, Georgia, to see Dr. Kolb, who works extensively with patients who have been exposed to toxins and has written several articles and books on the subject.

She looked at the reports and immediately knew the problem. The toxic chemical I was exposed to was mold, and there is hope for improvement and recovery. The mold has caused enough problems, and it has caused severe issues with my vision. How would the many neurologists feel if they had to spend two decades with a giant cobweb covering their thought process, visual, memory, concentration, and eye sockets?

It has taken years to get to the point of understanding the problem, and continually learning the healing process. There is never a point when I feel I have arrived on the toxic mountain of knowledge. I feel we always need to take an interest in our health because we are constantly bombarded with toxins from every direction, our surroundings, our food, lifestyle, and relationships. They are all important to living a long, healthy, happy, life.

I am going to devote one chapter to how I am detoxing because, for over two decades, I didn't know what toxins I was dealing with or that it was possible to remove them from my body. Now that I know how to detox and regain my health, I want to share the information so you don't need to spend years searching plus spending a ton of money in the wrong direction, like I did.

I am doing five things:

1. Toxicology Protocol Detoxification. Find a functional medicine doctor in your area so he or she can do muscle testing for toxins. Dr. Kolb put me on a detox program that I follow faithfully every day, but not everyone can afford to fly to Atlanta, so you need to find a functional doctor in your area. Dr. Kolb can be reached at www.plastikos.com, and she is a plastic surgeon and specializes in toxic chemicals and detoxification. She is also the author of *The Naked Truth about Breast Implants*. If you are in the Vineyard Haven, Massachusetts, area, Dr. Lisa Nagy is an environmental physician. Her website is www.lisanagy.com.

2. I purchased a BioMat for removing toxins and rebuilding my immune system. There is a chapter devoted to the Biomat. You can find out more at biomat4life.biomat.com

3. I started using Zeolite to remove toxins from my body. I spray it in my mouth three times a day.

4. I replaced all cleaning, body and hair and skin care products with chemical- free products. (The first thing I did that began the healing process. I have a chapter devoted to it). Thank You Melaleuca). Tell them you heard about it from me.

5. I also purchased a Shark steam cleaner. It cleans all of my floors including hardwood, tubs, sinks, counters, woodwork, blinds, windows, and showers with distilled water. It's easy to use and safe with absolutely no chemicals.

Check to see if there is an environmental doctor in your area if you have unusual symptoms, your symptoms mimic diseases, or you have an undiagnosed illness.

I absolutely love the BioMat, and I can feel a difference in two areas already. The quality of my sleep is so much better. I sleep without sleeping pills and earplugs. Plus, it is amazing how I have been able to relax. When you are constantly in pain and have health issues, your body is always on high alert waiting for the next attack. The BioMat gives you permission to relax for an hour while the negative ions and far infrared heat work to detox my body.

It's much better than several of the other things I tried over the years. Once I remember my good friend Darrel calling and telling me he bought a machine that he was sure would fix my problem, whatever it was. He said it looked like a space suit, and all I needed to do was put it on and zip it up so the only part of me sticking out of the suit was my head. Then I would put the tube attached to an ozone bottle into the suit, and ozone would fill the suit.

I followed the instructions explicitly, and thirty minutes later, I walked into the living room smelling like a chlorinated swimming pool. I used the ozone machine for a couple weeks, but every time I walked into a room, people would start sniffing because of the strange odor. Darrel suggested that, instead of using the suit, I just use the tube and put the ozone directly into my ears. That worked for another two weeks until my ears and head broke out in white bumps, which promptly ended my ozone therapy.

Another idea Darrel had for helping me regain my health and vitality was the fermented mushroom therapy. I made this ugly-looking mushroom, and first thing in the morning, I strained fermented mushrooms and drank the juice. I managed to stick with it for about two months before abandoning the idea.

Darrel went from mushrooms to the pasture. I had this really bad alfalfa-looking stuff that would do wonders. All I needed to do was mix it and drink it first thing in the morning. It made me want to stay in bed until noon.

I don't care how good something is supposed to be for you. If it tastes terrible, you won't stick to it.

Lessons I've Learned in My Life!

Remember, you don't need a certain number of friends ... just a number of friends you can be certain of.

Chapter 7 Review

1. Name four of the most common household toxins.

_____

_____

_____

_____

2. Name five of the eighteen listed symptoms of toxicity.

_____

_____

_____

_____

3. What are seven of the thirty symptoms of neurotoxicity?

1._____   2._____

3._____   4._____

5._____   6._____

7._____

8

IS THERE A BETTER, SAFER WAY?

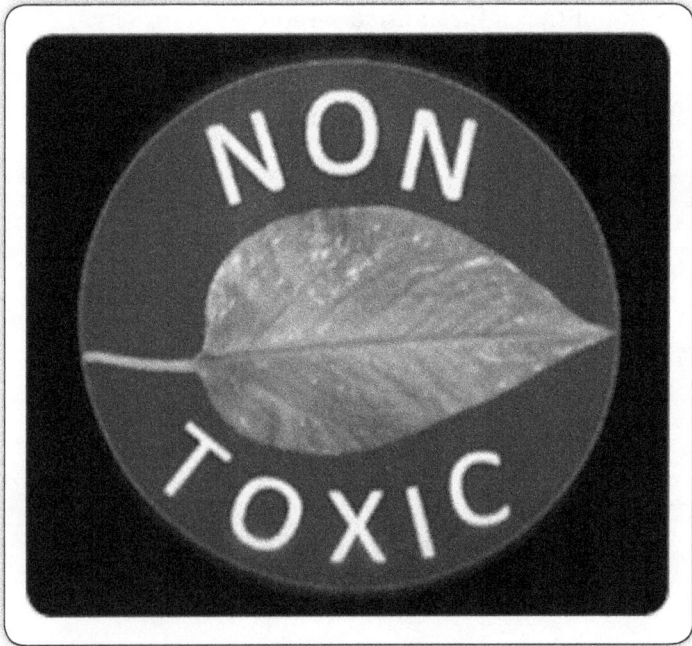

There are two primary choices in life: to accept conditions as they exist, or accept the responsibility for changing them.

http://izquotes.com/quote/191745

—Denis Waitley

Many of the chemicals found in our homes are used to make our lives easier. But we don't realize the consequences of using many of these substances. Think before you pour waste down the sink. Only natural substances should be disposed of in our sewer systems. Be wary and read labels, and the best decisions are to use alternative nontoxic products that will curtail the destruction of the environment.

Everyone is exposed on a daily basis, but if you are showing symptoms of chemical exposure, then it is better to be proactive rather than inactive. What you can do is follow the following sixteen steps to help limit your exposure.

- Only use chemical-free cleaning products in your home.

- Switch over to chemical-free toiletries.

- Get plenty of safe sun exposure to boost your vitamin D levels and your immune system (helping you to better fight disease).

- Have your tap water tested, and install an appropriate water filter on all your faucets (even those in your shower or bath) if contaminants are found.

- Read product labels. Don't use products that use the words *caution*, *danger*, or *keep out of reach of children*. If it says keep out of reach, find a chemical- free brand.

- Find and purchase cleaning solutions that bear the Green Seal logo.

- Interview cleaning services and hire one that is Green Clean Certified.

- The Green Seal certifies cleaning products are effective at cleaning yet safer for human health and the environment.

- Many national and local cleaning companies are now making the switch to green products, but you should ask exactly what they are using.

- Become an advocate for your own health and the health of your family.[8]

- Choose cleaners in the largest container sizes available. Especially look for bulk sizes to reduce packaging waste.

- Select products in bottles made with at least some recycled plastic, thus supporting companies that are providing a vital end market for recycled plastic.[9]

- Choose concentrated formulas that contain only 20 percent or less water.[10]

- When ingredients are listed, choose products made with plant-based—instead of petroleum-based—ingredients.

- Avoid products that list active ingredients of chlorine or ammonia, which can cause respiratory and skin irritation and will create toxic fumes if accidentally mixed together.

- Avoid cleaners marked danger or poison on the label, and look out for other telltale hazard warnings, such as "corrosive" or "may cause burns."

I found a company that could provide my toxic-free cleaning solutions along with my chemical-free body and hair care, medicine cabinet, cosmetic, and nutritional products.

- Without this market, recycling would not be possible.

- Because dilution with water is done at home, not at the factory, concentrated cleaners overall require less packaging and fuels for shipping.

- Look for a signal word on the product label, such as *danger*, *warning*, or *caution*, that provides some indication of a product's toxicity.

- Look for instructions on how to use the product that may help avoid injury.

Some labels do list active ingredients, which may assist you in detecting caustic or irritating ingredients you may wish to avoid, such as ammonia or sodium hypochlorite. A few manufacturers voluntarily list all ingredients.

Will it make a difference in your life if you remove toxic chemicals from your home and live a healthier lifestyle? You can be the judge. If you change to a chemical-free environment (at least at home) and you work on living a healthier lifestyle, will it make a difference? Absolutely! If you continue using products that have labels that read "Keep out of the reach of children" and most of your meals are processed foods, will it make a difference? Absolutely! You will probably cut your quality of life in half.

One person can make a difference. I read the story of Megan Rice who learned that her daughter's sippy cups contained BPA, which is linked to synthetic estrogen and a number of health problems. The manufacturers contend that it poses no health risk.

She immediately tossed them in the trash. She boarded a bus headed for Washington, DC, in May 2013, along

- with hundreds of moms and their strollers known as the "stroller brigade," delivering petition signatures to members of Congress demanding action on toxic chemicals. Never underestimate a band of women on a mission who have hundreds of voices that become a single, powerful voice.

We can't control all toxins that surround us, but *we can use common sense before we say yes to an elective surgery that may affect the rest of our life. Choose the products wisely that you inhale, ingest, and rub on your body.* And whatever you do, *don't buy your cleaning products at the grocery or dollar store.* You are saving pennies, and it may end up costing you millions or your life. *If you can't pronounce it and it requires a safety lock on your cupboards, you probably shouldn't have it.*

It isn't the number of breaths you take that is important. It is the number of moments that take your breath away that are important.

Make sure you have the time to enjoy the special moments in life and you are healthy so you can appreciate it.

Lessons I've Learned in My Life!

If you build your relationships around positive people, you will have a solid foundation.

Chapter 8 Review

1. Name six of the sixteen ways you can limit your exposure to toxic chemicals.

   _____

   _____

   _____

   _____

   _____

   _____

2. Make a list of ways you can start to improve the health and safety of your family.

Cleaning Products

   _____

   _____

   _____

Hair/Body Care

   _____

   _____

   _____

Cosmetics/Skincare

   _____

   _____

   _____

9

DETECTING AND DETOXING

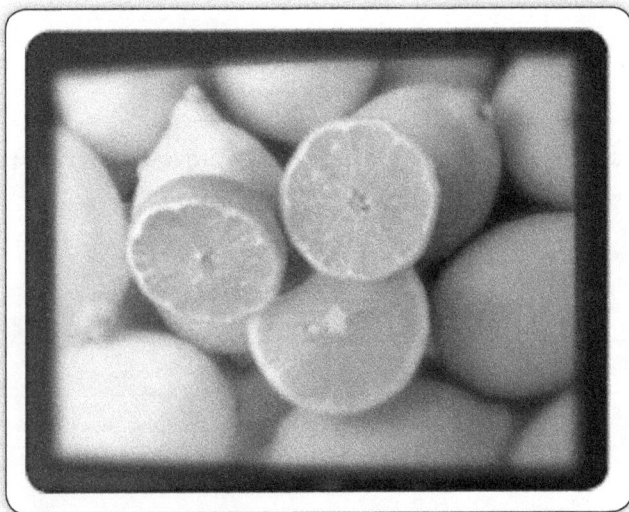

Detoxing entails getting the toxic contamination out of the body, but in addition, you must work on stopping the contamination sources. It is important to begin and work at restoring the body to regain your health, and while you will make great improvements, it is sometimes difficult to recover completely from chemical exposure. It depends on your dedication to work at it consistently.

Toxins kill body cells, and the cells that die will not come back to life; however, the toxins additionally alter the DNA of your cells. When you detox, not only do you remove toxins, you also stop continual destruction to your cells.

Next, I have provided some general guidelines to help you get started on your road to finding out why you are sick, what caused your illness, where to find help, and how to get on the road to recovery. This information will be based on my experience, plus my countless hours of research and the people I have met who have walked in your shoes. All of the advice is coming from people who had illnesses and symptoms that traditional medicine was not helping, so most of us had to strike out on our own. And along the way, our paths crossed, and we became friends. I hope our experience helps you as you travel in our footsteps. I am speaking based on my experience as a person with toxic chemical exposure. I am not a doctor, and I do not give medical advice.

If you have a mystery illness or you've been to a number of doctors and your health is not improving, maybe there is a reason. Most medical doctors don't know about toxic exposure. Medical schools generally don't teach classes on how toxins affect the human body. If they had classes, they may not prescribe medications as freely because that is only adding additional toxins to bodies that are in toxic overload. If you are planning to detox, you will be on your own for most of the work unless you find a functional medical doctor, environmental doctor, or naturopathic or homeopathic doctor.

The following is a brief roadmap to help you discover the cause of your toxic exposure and to show you basic detox steps.

Discovering the Cause

- Maintain a diary of symptoms.

- Note specific symptoms along with the time they occur.

- Notice the place you're at when symptoms begin, and write it down.

- Write down what you ate and the source of drinking water.

You're searching for a pattern. From the pattern, you might be able to uncover both the place making you sick and maybe the foods, issues, and locations to which you might have become allergic. Allergic reactions to foods develop when you find yourself poisoned, as the immune system (unable to discriminate between toxins and the foods combined with the toxins) learns to reject the contents that are present when toxins are present. Because the body absorbs toxins and stores them, the immune system activates the contaminated body substance, and the body becomes allergic to the contamination and autoimmune response. Disease begins. This is one way the disease process can activate illnesses or mimic them.

- Look for information from past records to find the previous timing of your symptoms.

- Take a look at time sheet information of time absent from school or work as a result of sickness or emergency room visits.

- Review information from physician visits and time without work as a result of fatigue.

- Look at canceled checks and telephone data, as this can jog your memory of the place you were whenever you got sick.

- Look at the over-the-counter or prescription medicine and treatment purchases.

- Make a journal of conversations you have had with friends and family members about your symptoms and illness.

- Write down dates of examinations and tests and results if available.

Uncover the symptoms Muscle spasms and cramps from pesticide exposure could be instant: however, it could also be a delayed response by as much as three days and even up to six weeks. Diarrhea typically begins inside ten minutes to a half hour after exposure and lasts a number of hours; however, it could start as much as three hours later if the exposure isn't severe. It's usually followed a day or more later with constipation and light-colored smelly bowel movements, along with other symptoms, if the toxins have killed the bowel flora.

Toxins may be obvious; however, they are usually not apparent. Even very small quantities can have an impact if you're exposed repeatedly or for an extended period of time. Toxins could also be much less apparent.

Toxins could be things like pesticides, gasoline, solvents, fragrance, carpet glue, shampoo, shaving cream, aftershave lotion, cosmetics, detergents, soaps, cleaning products, turpentine, mildew, bedding, industrial products, photographic items, mold, carpets, lotion, formaldehyde, dry-cleaned garments, and carbon monoxide.

In my case, I didn't have any symptoms for the first three months that I was aware of; however, when I realized there was a problem, it happened suddenly. From that point, I had continual pain and symptoms.

Some individuals have been exposed to chemical substances by repeated incidents of exposure, experiencing acute but passing flulike symptoms, fatigue, sore throat, upset stomach, fever, earache, and headache; however, they grew to become cumulatively sick and less capable of recovering.

With repeated exposure, a time comes when the chemical substances cling to the tongue, pervade the sinuses, and induce brain fog; dizziness; muscle ache; spasms; bone pain/ density loss; joint, back, wrist, or foot pain; numb extremities; fatigue; twitching eyelids; peripheral vision loss; night vision loss; earache; swollen interior ears; ear discharge; sore throat; swollen lymph nodes, stomach, head, or gums; tooth enamel erosion; deformed nails; lack of libido; impotence; cold fingers and toes; excess menstrual bleeding; endometriosis; sleep disturbance; failure to sweat; failure to moisturize mouth and throat, pores and skin, or eyes (alternating with extreme tearing); hair loss; constipation, smelly gas; failure to soak up vitamins from one's meals; incapacity to regulate one's internal thermostat; dark under-eye circles; and weakening, irregular heartbeat. These are a few of the varied symptoms of acute and cumulative toxic chemical exposure.

Toxic exposure affects each part of the body. At first, just a few of the symptoms might be observed; however, as the exposure continues without intervention, many will present themselves. Many different toxins have related effects. Many pharmaceuticals are the identical chemical substances and cause related effects.

This may be the reason why I had such a severe reaction to the drug Tegretol at Mayo Clinic two nights before leaving to return to Idaho. I would not have been able to get on my flight if it had not been for the kindness of strangers. The neurological symptoms were the worst they had been in years and lasted for almost two months.

The Importance of Heat

Detoxing requires heat, both internal and external. That is one more reason the BioMat in the next section is so effective.

Simple Ways You Can Detox on a Budget

When you detox, you may experience elimination symptoms that may not be pleasant but are necessary as part of the healing process. Symptoms may include headaches, muscle/joint aches and pains, diarrhea, fatigue, and weakness. You can help yourself by increasing your intake of distilled water and resting.

- **The Lemon Water-Cayenne-Maple Syrup Fast.** This will give your GI tract a rest, and it's a great short-term way you can go for a few days. This combination provides you with the liver-flushing power, energy, and minerals. Just make sure you gradually sequence into eating healthy foods by starting with easily digested organic produce.

- **Juicing Fast.** This also gives your GI tract a break from hard work to heal. If you have a blender, mix some organic veggies with greens and purified water. Then strain out the bulk fibers to make the solution totally liquid.

- **Heavy Metal Detoxing.** You can juice organic cilantro in a juicer or blender and add powdered chlorella (the least expensive form). Cilantro and chlorella actually chelate heavy metals, including mercury. You can also drink chlorella powder with water and lots of lime/lemon. Make sure you're drinking lots of water and eliminating thoroughly to prevent those heavy metals from relocating into other organs.

- **Apple Fasting Detox.** Eat only organic apples for three days while drinking lots of pure water. As an optional flush, the morning after, with an empty stomach, drink two ounces of fresh orange juice mixed thoroughly with an equal amount of castor oil for bowel flushing. Stay home and keep drinking water.

When I started searching earlier this year for ways to detox and remove the toxins from my body, I found so many ideas. I spent days going from one Google search to another. The problem was that I had already spent a fortune on doctors, tests, and prescription drugs, and we know that didn't work. By this time, I was very skeptical of what would work and what was just going to take my money with absolutely no results. The one thing I knew for sure was that now I was on the right path because I was surrounding myself with people who had walked this path and knew which road to take.

The blogs, websites, books, and resources were people who knew what they were talking about so I felt confident that I was spending my money wisely. I ran across a story about a young woman who developed multiple chemical sensitivities that came on slowly while working out at the gym. She finally stopped doing her cardio workout. Then she couldn't tolerate people's perfume, fabric softener, or deodorant until she finally had to give up going to the gym. Her friends thought she was neurotic, her doctors thought she was a hypochondriac, and of course, her family thought she was a recluse because she was afraid to go out of her house.

She studied everything she could about toxic chemicals and read many books, including most of the books written by Dr. Sherry Rogers, and she began detoxing in an effort to get well. Her regular doctor just looked at her with a blank stare like she was crazy when she told her about her daily detox regimen to get better. Next, she ignored her and then dropped her as a patient. She went to ten more doctors in an attempt to find a doctor who understood about multiple chemical sensitivities, but none of them knew or wanted to learn about it.

Because she spent hours at home alone, she had time on her hands to read books and research on the computer about multiple chemical sensitivities and how they affect your body. She started detoxing, improved her nutrition, cleared her home of all toxins, and got air and water purifiers. She also included acupuncture, nutritional supplements, and hot saunas.

The good news is, after about nine months of detoxing, her health started to improve, but she knew she needed to work at taking better care of her body every day. I am happy to report that I have been following her story, and over the past couple years, her health continues to improve. Everyone exposed to toxic chemicals may experience different symptoms, and your detox and healing may also be dissimilar as well.

What is important is that you are an active participant in maintaining your health, not a passive bystander.

I can't even begin to give you a quick, easy three-day or ten-day detox fix. Once you have reached toxic overload, you won't find a quick fix. You can improve your health and regain your vitality if you are willing to take the time and do the work. Most of us got ill to begin with because of either lack of knowledge or looking for an easier, simpler way to get a job done. We relied on the government to look after our product safety, along with the manufacturers, producers, pharmaceutical companies, or doctors when we had elective surgeries, and they said the product was safe.

Sometimes, we make a choice to buy a product that will make our life easier, but as it turns out, it isn't making our life easier because we are consuming more toxins daily than our bodies can handle, so we need to learn how to remove the toxins from our life. That is a tall order, but I am going to give you a starting point. Detoxing is more than a quick cleanse or buying a product. It is an ongoing lifestyle.

It begins with learning about ways to avoid toxins and discovering techniques to boost your whole body's health.

Ten Easy Steps to Remove Toxins from Your Body and Environment

1. Remove toxic chemicals and products from your home.

2. Avoid toxic and negative relationships. (If you hang out with positive people, you will have a healthy environment.)

3. Meditate daily. Meditation calms down your restless thinking and allows you to have control over your mind. It also frees your mind from negative thinking, worries, and unhappiness. Meditation improves the ability to focus the mind, think

more clearly, and have a clearer understanding of what you learn. It strengthens your intuition and develops the ability for constructive and creative thinking. It will also make you more patient, tolerant, and considerate and increase your inner strength.

4. Use a coffee enema to detox the liver, flush out yeast and toxins before they have a chance to reabsorb, and kill parasites. Use organic coffee, clean water, and nontoxic cookware (glass, ceramic, or stainless steel). Boil the water on the stove, and add the coffee. Strain. Don't put through your plastic coffee brewer. Use a stainless steel enema kit to avoid leaching toxins out of plastic.

5. Detox with a cocktail of vitamin C 2000, alpha lipoic acid 300, lipsomal, and glutithione 300 twice per day (recommended by Dr. Sherry Rogers in *Detoxify or Die*).

6. Use colonics to help clean toxins out of the colon. But they can get expensive. I try to get a series of five at least once a year.

7. Use acupuncture, which is based on the premise that there are patterns of energy flow (qi) through the body that are essential for health. Disruptions of this flow are believed to be responsible for disease.

8. Drink two quarts of water daily. Water is vital to every part of the body. Water in the blood helps to carry oxygen to the body's cells. Water also helps to digest food and rid the body of toxins.

9. Use saunas to stimulate the lymphatic system and move toxins that are trapped in fat. Start off with ten minutes and work up to three ten- to twenty- minute sessions. Infrared plug-in saunas emit EMFs, heat the brain, and only penetrate one to two inches into the body. Don't enter a sauna alone if you're in

an acute condition. Entry to a sauna is one option to start the process of detoxification. Along with entry to the sauna, you will want to have:

- Activated charcoal capsules from the health food store, capsules with 250– 380 milligrams each (helps mop up toxins from the blood)

- Non timed release niacin (100 milligrams at first)

- Timed release niacin (250 milligrams)

- About a half gallon of filtered water or more

- Entry to a bathroom

- Acidophilus/bifidous capsules

- Three or more twelve-ounce drinks each of 1000-milligram vitamin C crystals dissolved in water and a straw

- 300 milligrams of magnesium above normal supplements

10. Use additional herbs for detoxing. Molybdenum converts toxins from candida and parasites into energy. There are risks and side effects if not monitored and dosed correctly, so I am not recommending you start buying all of the herbs listed and just start taking them. The best way is to find the right type of doctor who understands the detox process. If you live in area that does not have a functional or environmental physician, then the following list can help get you started:

DHEA (many MCS people are deficient)	NAC (detoxifier)	Carnatine
Vitamin D (essential)	Iodine	Green Tea Extract
Milk Thistle (liver detoxifier)	Ginger	Wheat Grass Powder
Barley Grass Powder	CoQ10	Pomegranate Juice
Fresh Wheatgrass Juice	Milk Thistle	Blackberry Juice
Chlorella (heavy metal detoxifier)	Goji Berries	B Vitamins
Turmeric (anti- inflammatory/ anti- parasite)	Cysteine	Magnesium
Oregano (anti-allergy/yeast, Anti- fungal/bacterial)	Vitamin E	

Lessons I've Learned in My Life!

I've learned that, when you look at the big picture, it really doesn't matter if you use your stove as a filing cabinet and your pantry as a closet for your hats. What really matters the most is, "Are you happy?"

Chapter 9 Review

1. Discover the cause of your illness. (Use additional paper if necessary.)

Symptoms past/dates   **Symptoms/present**

_____

_____

_____

_____

_____

Medications past/dates   Medications present/dates

_____

_____

_____

_____

Labs/MRI/EEG/CAT/etc. past   **Labs/MRI/EEG/CAT/etc. present**

_____

_____

_____

_____

_____

_____

_____

_____

2. Name six of the twenty-four products that, if you were exposed to very small quantities repeatedly for a long time, would have an impact:

   1.   2

   3.   4.

   5.   6.

3. Name seven of the forty-three symptoms that you may experience with repeated exposure to toxic chemicals.

   1.   2

   3.   4.

   5.   6.

   7.

10

TOXIN-FREE REGAINING YOUR HEALTH

I think a hero is an ordinary individual who finds strength to persevere and endure in spite of overwhelming obstacles. http://chrisreevehomepage.com/

—Christopher Reeve

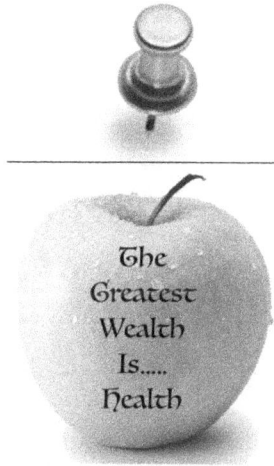

The
Greatest
Wealth
Is.....
health

It's impossible to avoid all environmental toxins. While I was doing the research for this book, I happened to find six products/companies that are worth mentioning that help remove toxic chemicals from the body and home and help you regain and maintain your health.

Health doesn't just happen.........We need to take responsibility for our health. Good health won't happen by accident. It will happen because we intentionally work toward the goal of a healthy lifestyle. Hopefully we don't just sit around and wait until we fall apart and then go to the medical team and expect them to put us back together. When the doctor puts us back together it will never be it the condition we dreamed about. It will usually be with stitches and prescriptions. Not the ideal lifestyle.

Melaleuca Is Committed to Superior Products: Every product has been developed and manufactured to stand out from the competition. Each must be superior in a very clear and relevant way to the products you might otherwise use. That means they are researched, refined, and scrutinized before they ever go to market. Melaleuca Preferred Members deserve only the best. And that is exactly what Melaleuca is committed to providing.

I wouldn't have been able to stabilize in my recovery and discover how to heal so quickly had it not been for this company. By removing all of the toxic substances from my environment all at once and replacing them with healthy eco-friendly products my body had the ability to heal little by little.

I have been symptom free for the same amount of time that I have been using these wonderful products. Both my body and my budget says "Thank You Melaleuca for helping me regain my life." Saving money meant nothing if I couldn't enjoy my life.

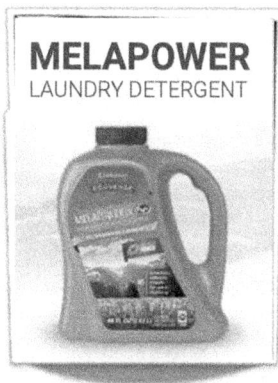

Melaleuca Products are SAFER for your **Home** and **Family** because the are environmental-friendly

No Bleach

No Ammonia

No Phosphates

The largest online wellness shopping club in North America..

Melaleuca products feature biodegradable ingredients like thyme oil to disinfect surfaces, citric acid to remove hard water stains, enzymes to clean dishes, and cleaners to gently release tough stains from laundry.

Bath & Body

Beauty

Essential Oils

Vitamins

Nutrition

Medicine Cabinet

Household

Here's just a small sample:

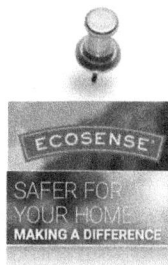

MELAPOWER
LAUNDRY DETERGENT

MelaPower 6x with Triple Enzyme Power has a super-concentrated, cost-saving, eco-friendly formula!

Trust MelaPower to keep your laundry, family, and world looking great—Because There's More Than Just Laundry on the Line.®

ECOSENSE

SAFER FOR YOUR HOME

MAKING A DIFFERENCE

SOL-U-GUARD
BOTANICAL DISINFECTANT

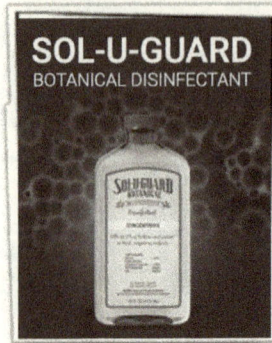

This one-of-a-kind EPA- approved botanical disinfectant combines thyme oil and citric acid, and kills 99.99% of germs.

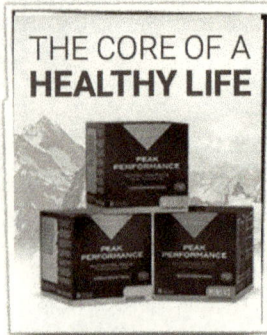

THE CORE OF A
HEALTHY LIFE

The *Peak Performance Pack* provides the vitamins and minerals you need every day to maintain a healthy lifestyle.*

SAFE & MIGHTY
TOILET BOWL CLEANER

An environmentally responsible and effective way to keep your toilet bowl clean and fresh. Contains no harsh chemicals and requires no child-proof caps.

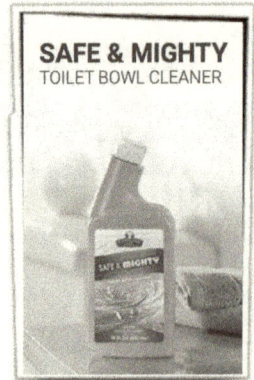

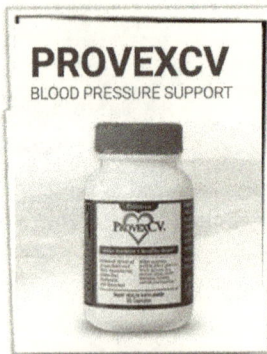

PROVEXCV
BLOOD PRESSURE SUPPORT

Helps maintain healthy blood pressure already in the normal range and promotes healthy endothelial function with a Patented blend that includes the antioxidant power of 10,000 grapes in every bottle

**PROVEN.
PROTECTED.
PATENTED.**

Proven by science to provide superior mineral absorption and minimize free radical damage.

Oligo

100 Years of Mineral Depletion since the industrialization of farming began more than a century ago the trace mineral content in fruits, vegetables, grains, meat, and dairy products has dropped precipitously. In the US, farmland mineral content has dropped more than 85%.

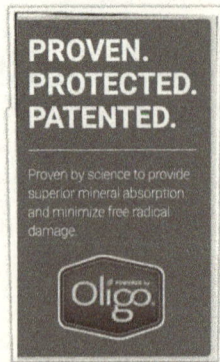

Higher Quality, Better Value
Solutions For Today's Major Health Concerns
Safer For Your Home
Better For The Environment
No Bleach No Ammonia No Phosphates

400 +

Products

Being a Melaleuca Preferred Member has its privileges. It introduces a new world of naturally effective, one-of-a-kind wellness products to you, your home, and your family. And with over 400 unique products to choose from, shopping with Melaleuca is always filled with variety and options.

Melaleuca Is Committed to Superior Products

- Every product has been developed and manufactured to stand out from the competition.

- Each must be superior in a very clear and relevant way to the products you might otherwise use.

- That means they are researched, refined, and scrutinized before they ever go to market.

- Melaleuca Preferred Members deserve only the best. And that is exactly what Melaleuca is committed to providing.

- Melaleuca only uses the best biodegradable ingredients!

- Using the very best natural ingredients from around the world, Melaleuca has developed a heart health system that is unrivaled.

- Safety caps aren't required!

- Melaleuca customers saved a total of 205 million pounds of plastic

- In addition Melaleuca Customers saved 41 million gallons of fuel

- And finally, Melaleuca customers saved 46 million pounds of harmful gas emissions

- You can find more information here: https://www.melaleuca.com. or contact a Melaleuca representative in your area.

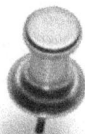

Toxic-Free Home

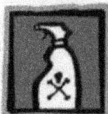 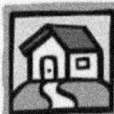 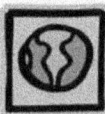

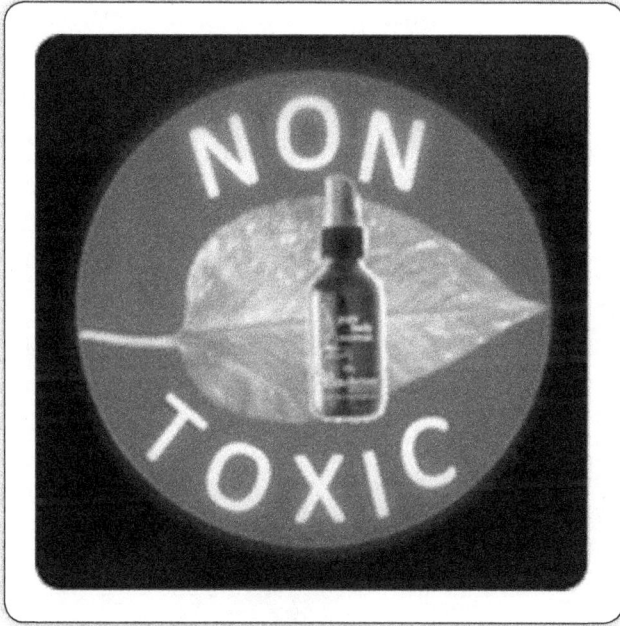

Zeolite Removes Toxins

Everyone is bombarded with toxic chemicals on a daily basis coming from different directions. We can wait until we are in crisis mode and look for solutions, or we can take control of our lives now and begin a healthier lifestyle. I would like to share a few ideas that are helping me achieve my goal of regaining my health. I found a company with an awesome product for removing toxins from the body: Pure Body Extra Strength.

Why detox? No matter how hard you try to minimize your exposure to chemicals and toxins, they keep showing up in our bodies in increased levels, simply because they are everywhere in our environment.

According to CDC reports, the average person now has 212 environmental chemicals in his or her blood, things like mercury, lead, cadmium, and plastic byproducts, which simply aren't supposed to be there.

Fortunately, nature provides protection against many of the toxic elements we encounter every day in the form of a natural mineral, zeolite. The zeolite clinoptilolite—a negatively charged mineral—works like a magnet, attracting positively charged toxins and safely and gently carrying them out of the body within hours.

Signs of chronic low-dose toxic exposure include feeling tired or lethargic, poor sleep quality, weight gain struggles, frequent headaches, and much worse. Rather than treating the symptoms of toxic overload, why not remove the source? With the proprietary processed zeolite, it is possible.

The Pure Body product line is carefully formulated to bind to positively charged heavy metals, radioactive particles, and VOCs. Pure Body's zeolite liquid concentrate provides a systemic and digestive detox, while Pure Body Extra Strength's spray features proprietary technology that amplifies detoxification for a powerful cellular cleanse.

Numerous studies attest to the selective nature of clinoptilolite to remove only toxins (and not good nutrients), and this zeolite is granted GRAS (generally recognized as safe) status by the FDA.

Pure Body is part of a line of products from Touchstone Essentials. I take zeolite three times a day to help remove the toxic chemicals from my body. Among the chemicals that zeolite removes are aluminum, lead, mercury, cadmium (highly toxic), arsenic, radioactive metals, nitrosamines, BPA, toulene, benzene, pesticides, and herbicides.

BioMat Healing Mat Removes Toxins

In January 2013, while researching my book, I met a nurse who believes that she had reversed early breast cancer and Lyme disease through her treatments on the BioMat. I tried it, and the first time I used it, I slept through the entire night peacefully. I am using it to detox my body.

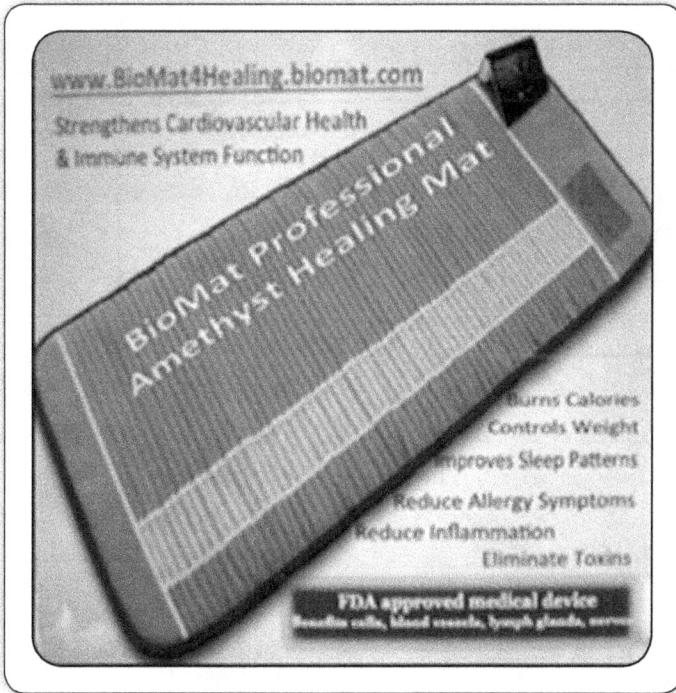

I introduced you to Janis earlier when she told her story about exposure to toxins and Lyme disease. The part of the story that she didn't share in that chapter was how she is improving her health.

Janis's Story

I contracted Lyme disease and some of the co-infections of Lyme in my childhood or early teens. I remember having the most horrific knee pains that would hit out of the blue, and I literally couldn't move during those episodes. I was sickly and had lots of medical issues, but I was not diagnosed with Lyme until I was in my mid-fifties. I am now sixty-one years old. I never really got treated because, even though I eventually saw a couple of the top Lyme doctors, I was faced with the overwhelming financial burden of the costly treatments and the havoc that years of antibiotics and other drugs would do to my body.

I tried some conventional treatments, but the side effects were unbearable, and I was unable to function. I felt utter despair and hopelessness with the financial burden for the treatments and also the degree of suffering. I chose to do supplements and just get by as best as I could. Many times, I wondered how I would live into old age and be able to bear all the suffering. I had no quality of life. I had wasted thousands of dollars seeing doctors, even flying to other states to see doctors always with the promise of hope, which would quickly fade. It was only through my faith in God that I was able to get through life.

My health was very unstable. I never knew from day to day how I would be. Sometimes I was in a wheelchair. Occasionally, I was bedridden and unable to care for myself. Other times, I seemed normal. I was in and out of the hospital and always had lots of medical bills. I started falling down and even broke my nose. I had a head/neck injury falling into a bed of rocks, along with other falls and injuries.

Early in 2012, I visited a local clinic for a ten-day cleansing program with daily colonics, a liver/gallbladder cleanse, and daily BioMat sessions. During my ten- day program, the best part was using the BioMat. I found that it relieved my pain and put me into a deep state of relaxation, which is a miracle as I am never relaxed or free of pain. I had a major flare-up of the Lyme disease after the liver/gallbladder cleanse as my liver has multiple cysts from the infections, and that really stirred things up. Shortly after I got home from the clinic, I could hardly walk or get in and out of a chair or the bed. My knees were swollen to twice their size. I was in pain from head to toe. I was utterly miserable!

In April 2012, I purchased the professional BioMat, pillow, and the Mini-Mat because I knew that, in order to kill Lyme and other organisms, I needed to be sandwiched between the two mats. As an RN and medical researcher, I had spent years researching my disease, and I knew the organisms did not like heat. In fact, Lyme disease is notorious for lowering the body temperature so it can survive and thrive. I had moved from San Diego to Idaho and gotten much worse when I moved to a cold climate. Those organisms were really thriving in Idaho. I just came back from seeing the holistic doctor who is able to give me a number through kinesiology testing of what my total body burden is with the Lyme disease. On February 15, 2011, my number was 990. And then in early 2012 (after the cleanse program), it was off the charts. He couldn't give me a number because it was higher than his reading goes. On June 5, 2012, my number was down to 790. Today, February 19, 2013, it is down to 440.

I have not being doing any real Lyme treatments, natural or conventional. I do take supplements but nothing specific to Lyme disease. I do the BioMat sessions almost daily at the highest heat setting (158) for thirty to sixty minutes. So it really seems it is killing off the Lyme organisms, not just improving my symptoms. I am so thrilled that this is really doing what I had hoped it would do. I know I feel better and have had no flares and hospitalizations. I've had much improved sleep and lowered pain, but to find out my numbers are dropping made my day.

If you lie on the full-length BioMat Professional, you will instantly feel the warmth of the infrared rays deeply penetrating your body as the negative ions deliver healing signals to every cell in your body. Because the BioMat's unique technology penetrates at the cellular level, it is capable of addressing a wide range of health issues. As well as providing relief from muscle and joint pain, the BioMat can also speed the repair and regeneration of these areas in the body. The BioMat also regulates the body's immune, endocrine, lymphatic, and nervous systems, delivering a wealth of health benefits, including improved cardiovascular strength; resilience to disease; deeper, more refreshing sleep; cellular detoxification; increased energy and focus; and more.

The BioMat's unique medical and therapeutic properties are based on Nobel prize–winning research into ionic channels and the same infrared technology that NASA identified as the safest and most beneficial type of light wave. By producing deep-penetrating, far infrared rays along with negative ions that activate the body at the molecular level, the BioMat is capable of administering deep stimulation and healing.

The Richway Amethyst BioMat Professional is an amazing healing tool that has changed thousands of lives for the better. Its most important function is to produce far infrared rays of light that penetrate six to seven inches deep into the body, warming all the cells and tissues evenly throughout. Rows of amethyst crystals that cover the entire surface of the BioMat produce these rays. The body experiences far infrared rays differently from other types of heat.

The BioMat Pro is highly recommended for both professional and home use. It is especially recommended when the goals of treatment are whole body in nature, such as strengthen cardiovascular health, promote general health maintenance, strengthen immune system function, relieve chronic and acute pain, burn calories/control weight, induce detoxification, improve sleep pattern, support core body temperature, reduce allergy symptoms, improve circulation, induce lymphatic drainage, and reduce inflammation. It is also an FDA-approved medical device.

The BioMat: Explanation of Technology
Far Infrared Light

This is light that is below the visible part of the spectrum. It penetrates several inches into most objects, transferring heat very efficiently. It is why sunlight feels warm. In comparison, heat transferred merely by conduction (contact) or convection (air flow) does not heat an object deeply or evenly throughout.

Negative Ions

These are particles in the air that have an extra electron. They are significant because bodies can be damaged by oxidative stress (free radicals), but breathing these free electrons neutralizes oxidizing compounds. Negative ions are an antioxidant. You may notice benefits of improved mood and alertness as well due to increased serotonin levels.

Amethyst

This material was chosen primarily because it converts heat energy into far infrared light very efficiently due to its crystalline structure. But its long use in the spiritual healing field across different cultures suggests it may have some more mysterious benefits as well. It has been called nature's superconductor.

The BioMat is designed to emit light at wavelengths that have healing properties. Amethyst was chosen because of its unique light signature and conductive properties. When heated, it emits light at eight and twelve microns of wavelength. This light, on the far infrared side of the spectrum, penetrates deeply into tissues, increases circulation and metabolism, and relieves pain directly.

Cells are able to absorb more oxygen, export more acidic wastes, and repair themselves faster when metabolism is higher. The healing tools have been found to benefit the treatment of chronic pain conditions, as well as autoimmune conditions, including fibromyalgia, back pain, neuropathy, Lyme disease, and even arthritis.

BioMat Aids and Supports Detox Process

When you hear the word *detox*, you might think about a detox from alcohol, cigarettes, or other commonly recognized addictive substances, but in fact, there are many toxic substances in your daily life—everything from the air you breathe to the plastics you eat and drink out of to the household cleaners you use to the stress and tension that accumulates in your body. Modern life is actually pretty toxic, which is why regular detoxing is so important to your health, vitality, and longevity.

The good news is that there are a variety of ways that you can detox, including healthy eating and hydration, retreats, yoga, meditation, and exercise classes. The BioMat is an ideal all-natural complement to any detox program.

The BioMat and Detoxification

The BioMat is an actual mat that uses advanced energetic technology to combine far infrared rays, negative ion therapy, and the amazing powers of pure amethyst crystals to promote healing and detoxification. Put simply, it gives your body a detox boost.

Its deep-penetrating heat stimulates cell repair and regeneration deep within the body, which can help you heal from illness, boost your energy and metabolism, soothe aching joints and muscles, restore overall body balance, help you sleep better at night, and remove toxins from the body. The BioMat increases circulation and stimulates the sweat glands by raising body temperature, helping the body release toxins and waste materials, including heavy metals, cholesterol, and more. All of this improves the immune system and helps you feel better and live healthier.

The BioMat is an FDA-registered class II medical device and has passed rigorous safety testing in order to be approved for use in hospitals, clinics, and home. The BioMat is very easy to use, and you can customize its settings to your detox needs and your schedule. Simply by resting on the BioMat for a short session of between fifteen and forty-five minutes, you can dramatically increase your body's natural detox capabilities and benefit from a wide range of health benefits.

Viruses prefer and promote a cold environment and replicate at a much more rapid rate when the body is cold. Viruses are killed and maintaining a warm body impedes further replication. Some bacteria such as Lyme spirochetes also prefer and promote a cold environment and can remain in a chronic state as long as a cold environment is maintained. Therefore, in the interest of the prevention and treatment of any viral, bacterial, or chronic illness, this topic must be understood.

The ultimate body coldness is seen in death. When observing a corpse many clinical gems can be gleaned and correlated to degenerative states of human suffering. In death, the blood and lymph fluid of the body solidify and the body becomes stiff and cold. In the same way, with many chronic cold illnesses, such as fibromyalgia, chronic fatigue, cancer, Lyme disease, multiple sclerosis, diabetes, and heart disease, we see that the body becomes progressively colder. As the body cools, the electrical oscillations of the fluids in the body slow down and there is a shift in the body's polarity, which promotes infectious microbes and cancer.

Low body temperature must be addressed to bring the body back to balance. The temperature must be elevated to end the dying process of the body and to help the body eliminate the cellular debris or the "sludge" in the body.

I am a certified hypnotherapist and also a customer of the BioMat Corporation. I immediately noticed the benefit of using the product in my hypnotherapy practice. I am also a distributor for the BioMat Corporation so that I can help my clients purchase any products they many need that I use in my practice.

To find out more about the BioMat go to: www.biomat4healing. biomat.com

The fourth product that I found that I feel is important for maintaining your heath is the Lifetime Vibe. The reason for this products is that over the years I have found that most of the people with health challenges don't have the energy or the desire to exercise but their body desperately needs it. So I was very impressed when my brother introduced me to the inventor of this product.

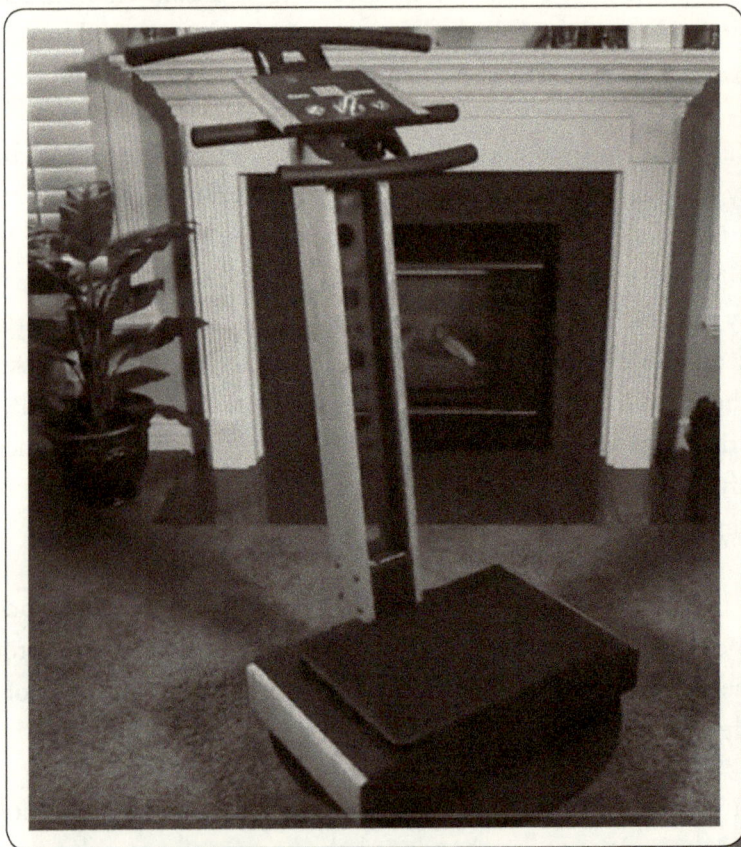

What does the Lifetime Vibe Do?

Whole Body Vibration is an innovative, safe, and effective exercise option. It is the use of a moving platform at specific frequencies and amplitudes to superimpose vibration on normal functional strengthening exercises. Like no other exercise, whole body vibration works directly through the nervous system creating a significant increase in the normal physiological responses of the body to exercise.

What makes the Lifetime Vibe Different?

Ten minutes on the Lifetime Vibe equals an hour of any other type of exercise. Even if you are in a wheelchair you are still able to use the Lifetime Vibe.

Who can use the Lifetime Vibe?

Whole Body Vibration is being used in hospitals, physical therapy clinics, and rehabilitation facilities. People who use this technology vary from the elderly, the person with physical disabilities, athletes who want to start to rehab an injury earlier, or just the general person looking to get toned and fit.

Is this a good product for Senior Citizens?

There are many factors that go with aging. Inactivity and stress are two. This exercise takes 10-20 minutes a day, at least three times per week. Vibration exercise has been shown to decrease the stress hormone cortisol and increase serotonin (a well-known contributor to feelings of well-being). If you have a feeling of well-being and you have muscle strength and balance you naturally have a joy in living. This promotes anti-aging.

How does gravity affect Whole Body Vibration?

Whole Body Vibration uses the power of gravity (the pull that is exerted by the earth). As the machine accelerates, it pushes up against your body and creates an extra force-known as a g-force. Imagine you were to hold a 12-pound weight in your hand. No problem right? Now imagine someone were to drop that weight, just by an inch or two, into your hand. You would have to use a little more strength to keep that weight from falling. The weight hasn't changed, but it feels heavier. Now, imagine someone were to drop that weight into your hand 30 times a second! Your muscles would be working much harder than if they were just holding the weight. So while your muscles are working to keep you balanced, they actually have to stabilize a heavier load than they would if you were standing on the ground. Your body literally feels as though it weighs more, meaning you have to work against an increased weight or "load" than your muscles are used to. Thus you are using the "POWER OF GRAVITY" to enhance your workout.

Will whole body vibration improve my flexibility?

Yes, this is one of the first things you will notice. Your body is becoming more flexible and your range of motion is increasing. Research has shown that stretch positions with vibration training will give an even greater increase in flexibility. An extra bonus is that your muscles are stretched in the same position as in everyday movement. Whole body vibration works your muscles by gently forcing the muscle to contract and release. This lengthens the fibers of your muscles, in other words, it stretches them as the muscle lets go.

Who is the ideal client the Lifetime Vibe?

The Lifetime Vibe is good for everyone, even athletes due to the lymphatic stimulation and the fact that it is is easy on your joints. Additionally, our research has found the follow people best benefit from this exercise:

1. Geriatric/Aging Boomers for balance, bone density, muscle stimulation, mood improvement through serotonin.

2. Athletes who want to improve core muscle function, extremity (foot/ankle) stabilization, and overall body awareness (Mechanoreceptors from joints, ligaments, muscles, and tendons aid in body orientation and Proprioceptors, which provide the sense of position).

3. Busy Executives use it for compressed time commitment. It is ideal for busy professionals who sit most of the day.

4. Travelers and long haul truck drivers. Sitting for long periods frequently can cause blood clots or other problems, which this can prevent.

5. New mothers/post pregnancy because certain postures will focus on strengthening and reducing around the hips, thighs and abdomen areas very quickly.

6. Back patients use whole body vibration because it is proven to actually help with many lower back issues.

A Few Conditions That Have Benefited from the Benefits Of The "Lifetime Vibe"

Arthritis	Cystic Fibrosis	Diabetes
Constipation	Fibromyalgia	Hip Pain
Fatigue	Cellulite	Dizziness
Incontinence	Insomnia	Knee Pain
Low Back Pain	Lymphatic System	Mobility
Multiple Sclerosis	Muscle Strength	Neck Pain
Neuropathy	Osteoporosis	Parkinson's Disease
Poor Circulation	Stress	TMJ
Weight Loss		

To find more about the Lifetime Vibe go to:
www.lifetimevibe.com/braintrainer
Enter code braintrainer to receive a discount.

The next product life changing product is…..ASEA

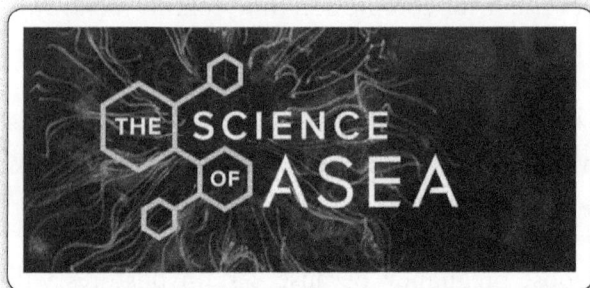

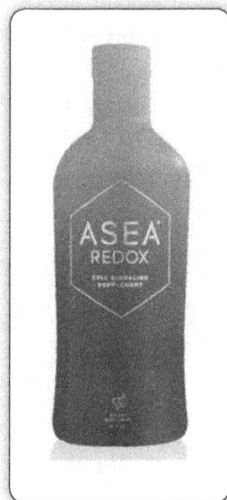

THE REDOX BREAKTHROUGH—Redox signaling is vital to strengthening the genetic signal that keeps our cells talking.

ASEAs breakthrough redox signaling technology provides critical connection and communication between cells to ensure optimal renewal and revitalization, supporting the development of new, healthy cells in the body.

ASEA REDOX Cell Signaling Supplement is a first-of-its-kind supplement that contains active redox molecules—cellular messengers that affect genetic expression in a positive way, helping to protect, rejuvenate, and keep cells functioning at optimal levels.

ANTIOXIDANTS—The test indicated that exposure to ASEA REDOX did cause a marked increase in antioxidants without invoking an inflammatory response.

Researchers found an 800% increase in effectiveness of glutathione after long exposure to ASEA REDOX.

ASEA:

- Improves immune system health
- Helps maintain a healthy inflammatory response
- Helps maintain cardiovascular health and support arterial elasticity
- Improves gut health and digestive enzyme production
- Modulates hormone balance to support vitality and wellness.
- More Energy
- Better Concentration
- Greater Vitality

ASEA is absorbed quickly through the channels in the soft tissues o the mouth, esophagus, and stomach lining.

The key to HEALTH begins at the cellular level.....CELLULAR HEALTH FROM THE INSIDE OUT! The key lies in how well out cells function.

Redox Signaling=cellular messages that help protect, invigorate and restore cells.

ASEA REDOX MOLECULES

I would like to share a story about someone I met through a leads program. She had since become a very dear friend. I was contacting her because I was looking for people that might be interested in starting a business with Asea.

During our conversation she mentioned her Dad was in the hospital and she wasn't she if he was going to live because he had so many health challenges.

I shared the ASEA story with her and I suggested she get a couple of bottles and try it and see how it worked for him. I did mention that since he was in the hospital she would need to sneak it into his room because if you ask the Doctor or nurse if it was ok to give it to him they would probably reject the idea. She had been a Nurse so I wasn't telling her anything she didn't already know so she ordered in the ASEA and her mother and her began giving Dad the Redox Molecules. Within a couple of days he was sitting on the edge of the bed, in another couple of days he was walking around the room and a week later he was released to go home. Lisa is thrilled that she has her Dad back and she is now part of the ASEA family and also responsible for sending me my final miracle product that is helping me and so many other people.

"The Jing Orb"

The final very impressive product with great results is "The Jing Orb." What is so impressive about this product? It works on the cellular level…..If you have the ability to heal at the cellular level…..the entire body will work more efficiently.

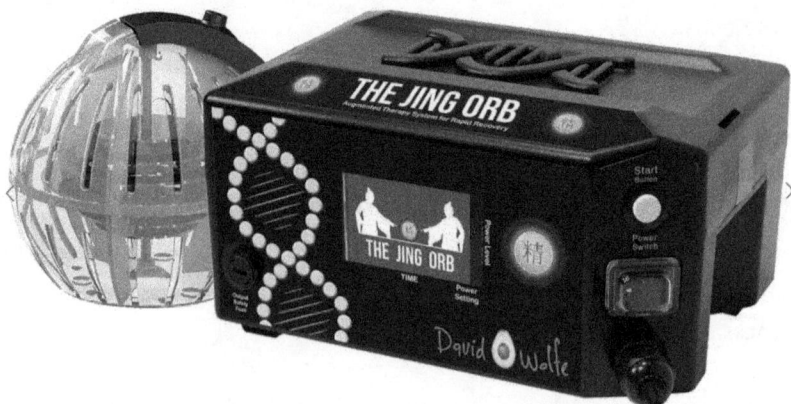

Each cell of our body contributes its part to our wellness. If they don't have the right charge, they can't perform their job properly. If too many cells are not performing correctly, then we start having health problems. By *restoring the cellular charge* to the right level, each cell is empowered to perform at its best, and that includes detecting and repairing damage.

Our body is made up of trillions of cells...about 75 *trillion* of them! Under ideal conditions, they all perform their job and are quite capable of detecting any damage that happens to them. Once damage is detected the cell knows to repair the damage. If that isn't possible, the cell is designed to literally self-destruct so that it can be replaced by a healthy cell. This process of repairing or replacing damaged cells is the very basis of the healing!

What is so exciting about "The Jing Orb?"

The Jing Orb (TJO) is a breakthrough health technology designed to recharge your body's biological batteries to promote overall wellness. To understand how the TJO works, think of each cell in your body as a miniature battery... and just like batteries, when your cells don't have enough charge, they don't function at optimal capacity.

Which is where TJO technology comes in.

By using the TJO you are boosting and topping off the charge on every cell! What's more, it's easy to use. You can have your whole body or just your hands and feet immersed in the water to get the benefits realized from using the device. The TJO can be experienced in your own home, office, spa, or patient practice.

So, you want the healthiest cells possible.
And TJO makes that possible.

When we are young our body is constantly replacing cells with healthy cells. That is why we naturally heal so quickly when we are little. Imagine what the impact would be as adults!

One of the stories related to "The Jing Orb" that I will share is about a woman that was in a serious auto accident. She received a severe back injury and the doctors said it would be several months before she would be able to walk again.

Her husband took her home from the hospital and he used "The Jing Orb" and within a week she was walking and before long she had regained her health.

The body is amazing! It has the capability to rejuvenate and heal if we give it the right tools but we abuse it day in and day out by the decisions we make.

It isn't easy to be healthy when we use toxic products, eat unhealthy and toxic food, lather toxic products on our body, and hang out with toxic people.

When an "Everyday Miracle" happens and someone tells us about a product that can make a real difference in our life I find that sometimes we ignore the life changing miracle and continue down the familiar path and our health doesn't improve. If I had not taken many chances over the years and ventured away from traditional medicine I probably would not be here to write this book. I decided to take responsibility for my own "health management" instead of letting the doctors control my "disease management" with drugs.

Just remember......**If a person or a book comes into your life.......
they are there for a reason........you might want to pay close
attention.....to a potential miracle.**

What are a few of the benefits of developing Healthy Cells?

Enhanced	Reduced
Moods	Stress, Anxiety, Hostility
Energy	Scars from Burns & Scalds
Stamina	Muscle Discomfort
Strength	Menstrual Discomfort.
Metabolism	Joint Discomfort.
Perception	Varicose Veins.
Concentration	Spider Veins.
Recovery Rate.	Fluid Retention.
Sleeping Patterns	Inflammation.
Meridian Balance.	Swelling.
Skin Rejuvenation and so much more	Cramping

When we are children our body is constantly replacing non-working and damaged cells with healthy cells. That is why we naturally heal so quickly. Imagine the impact if we had that same ability as adults and senior citizens.....Now it is possible!

If you want more information go to http://www.jingorb.com?ref=1120

Chapter 10 Review

The CDC has reported the average person has approximately environmental chemicals in their blood. _____.

The Pure Body Zeolite removes twelve different chemicals from the body. What are they?

1.   2

3.   4.

5.   6.

What are the three technologies that make up the BioMat?

1.

2.

3.

The BioMat Pro is highly recommended for the treatment of what conditions? (name at least 6)

1.   2

3.   4.

5.   6.

Which of the five products helped a woman in an auto accident who doctors said she would not be able to walk for months, was able to walk within a week?

_____

What product is the best product if you want to improve your balance?

_____

If you have allergies and sensitivities and the doctor has said you should find products that don't have perfumes and chemicals in them what company is worth considering from chapter ten?

Which product is designed to re-charge the cells of your body?

Name two products that will benefit you if have been diagnosed with the

following: Cancer   Multiple Sclerosis   Parkinson's Disease.
Inflammation   Insomnia   Energy.
1.
2.

Which of the five products is registered as a FDA medical devise?

Name three of the six ideal Lifetime Vibe clients?

1.

2.

3.

Name five of the twenty-five conditions listed that the Lifetime Vibe has helped.

1.

2.

3.

4.

5.

All six companies have life changing products and you can buy directly from the manufacturer. All it requires is a desire to have a better quality life. Some people spend their money on toys that lose value and break. If you don't have a family to take care of you, or you don't want to burden them, you need to learn how to take care of your body. Today's lifestyle is not healthy. It comes with a heavy price.

But we also have options that will help us as we journey to a healthy lifestyle but it require that we open our hearts and minds to what is available...... "Life is not measured by the number of breaths we take but by the moments that take our breaths away" **Miracles are all around us**

11

FINDING THE RIGHT DOCTOR

If you have been to several traditional doctors, you've been through tests and exams, and you still have symptoms along with prescriptions and a vague or undiagnosed problem, maybe you should look in a different direction. Traditional medical doctors normally do not test for toxic chemical exposure. They didn't even do it when I told them what I thought my problem was.

I was never tested until I flew from Idaho to California to a special lab to have the tests performed. I was right. I had a problem with toxic chemicals, but when I brought the results back to my home state, I still couldn't find a doctor who would treat my problem. My doctors were treating my symptoms, but I really needed someone to treat my entire body without using prescription drugs. I needed to change my thinking on the type of doctor who could treat my condition, which meant I also needed to be open-minded to all possibilities, not just traditional doctors.

It took me twenty years to find what I needed, but you will be able to find what you desire at the click of a button.

What Is Functional Medicine?

> We need to listen to the patient's story and develop a response to it. The approach to complex syndromes

may be much more profound than just trying to point a round peg into a square hole and get a singular diagnosis.

—Jeffrey S. Bland, PhD, the pioneer of functional medicine http:// www.jeffreybland.com

Functional medicine addresses the underlying causes of disease using a systems- oriented approach and engaging both patient and practitioner in a therapeutic partnership. It is an evolution in the practice of medicine that better addresses the health-care needs of the twenty-first century. By shifting the traditional disease- centered focus of medical practice to a more patient-centered approach, functional medicine addresses the whole person, not just an isolated set of symptoms. Functional medicine practitioners spend time with their patients, listening to their histories and looking at the interactions among genetic, environmental, and lifestyle factors that can influence long-term health and complex, chronic disease. In this way, functional medicine supports the unique expression of health and vitality for each individual.

Why Do We Need Functional Medicine?

- Our society is experiencing a sharp increase in the number of people who suffer from complex, chronic diseases such as diabetes, heart disease, cancer, mental illness, and autoimmune disorders like rheumatoid arthritis.

- The system of medicine practiced by most physicians is oriented toward acute care, the diagnosis and treatment of trauma or illness that is of short duration and in need of urgent care, such as appendicitis or a broken leg. Physicians apply specific, prescribed treatments such as drugs or surgery that aim to treat the immediate problem or symptom. Unfortunately, the acute care approach to medicine lacks the proper methodology and tools for preventing and treating complex, chronic disease. In most cases, it does not take into account the unique genetic makeup of each individual or factors such as environmental exposures to toxins and the aspects of today's lifestyle that have a direct influence on the rise in chronic disease in modern Western society.

- There's a huge gap between research and the way doctors practice. The gap between emerging research in basic sciences and integration into medical practice is enormous—as long as fifty years—particularly in the area of complex, chronic illness.

- Most physicians are not adequately trained to assess the underlying causes of complex, chronic disease and to apply strategies such as nutrition, diet, and exercise to both treat and prevent these illnesses in their patients.

How Is Functional Medicine Different?

Functional medicine involves understanding the origins, prevention, and treatment of complex, chronic disease. Hallmarks of a functional medicine approach include:

- **Patient-centered care.** The focus of functional medicine is on patient-centered care, promoting health as a positive vitality beyond just the absence of disease. By listening to the patient and learning his or her story, the practitioner brings the patient into the discovery process and tailors treatments that address the individual's unique needs.

- **An integrative, science-based health-care approach.** Functional medicine practitioners look "upstream" to consider the complex web of interactions in the patient's history, physiology, and lifestyle that can lead to illness. The unique genetic makeup of each patient is considered, along with both internal (mind, body, and spirit) and external (physical and social environment) factors that affect total functioning.

- **An integration of best medical practices.** Functional medicine integrates traditional Western medical practices with what is sometimes considered *alternative* or *integrative* medicine, creating a focus on prevention through nutrition, diet, and exercise—for example, use of the latest laboratory testing and other diagnostic techniques and prescribed combinations of drugs and/or botanical medicines, supplements, therapeutic diets, detoxification programs, or stress management techniques. For more information, you can contact http://www.functionalmedicine.org

Environmental Medicine

The mission of environmental medicine is to increase the understanding of the health risks posed by contaminants at home, in the workplace, and in the ambient environment and give solutions to lower client risks. In addition, environmental medicine emphasizes the relationship of health and disease to environmental factors. Diagnosis and treatment is directed at determining the cause of the illness. Through investigation, a determination is made of the correlation of the patient's disease process to environmental factors.

The mission is to provide in-depth, effective medical care and education, which treats the cause of illness and enables the patient to understand and become proactive in the healing process. You will receive a blend of traditional and alternative as part of your treatment; however, the therapies that are generally part of the treatment include sauna or other heat therapy, detox, massage, vitamin and mineral replacement, immunotherapy, patient education, nutrition and nutritional tests, exercise, osteopathic manipulation, and elimination or rotation diets.

Among the areas of specialty are implant syndrome, neurotoxicity, cardiovascular disease, mold exposure, vasculitis, immune dysregulation, IBS, metal toxicity, nutritional imbalances, chemical exposure, autoimmune disorders, fibromyalgia, chronic infections, thyroid disorders, ADD/ADHD, and sensitivities to EMF, chemicals, mold, dental materials, metals, foods, medications, surgical procedures, pollen, dust, and dust mites.

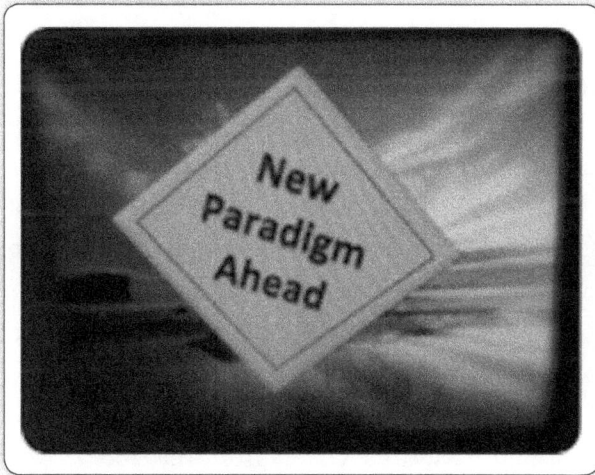

Alternative Medicine

Alternative medicine is any of a wide range of health-care practices, products, and therapies using methods of medical diagnosis and treatments, which, at least up to the end of the twentieth century, were typically not included in the degree courses of established medical schools teaching medicine, including surgery.

Examples include homeopathy, Ayurveda, chiropractic, and acupuncture.

Complementary medicine is alternative medicine used together with conventional medical treatment in a belief, not proven by using scientific methods, that complements the treatment. CAM is the abbreviation for Complementary and Alternative Medicine. Integrative medicine (or integrative health) is the combination of the practices and methods of alternative medicine with evidence-based medicine.

The term *alternative medicine* is used in information issued by public bodies in the United States of America and the United Kingdom. Regulation and licensing of alternative medicine and health-care providers varies from country to country and state to state.

Chiropractic

We have the most amazing healing power inside of our bodies. This healing power is called the nervous system. It is made up of the brain, spinal cord, and nerves. In order for us to be healthy and able to detox properly, the healing power must go from our brain, down the spinal cord, and out the nerves to every single organ, cell, and tissue. This system is so important that it is the only system in the body completely enclosed in bone. In order to be healthy, the spine needs to be straight from the front and have three curves from the side. If we lose one of these normal curves or even one bone shifts out of position, it will cause problems throughout the whole body called a subluxation.

Not only does subluxation cause pain, the body becomes out of balance, which leads to problems with detoxing and developing disease within the body.

Subluxation is what corrective care chiropractors analyze and correct. Not only does chiropractic help remove aches and pains, it also helps your body function better so it can detox and heal. Corrective care chiropractors correct the spine and keep you straight from the front. A chiropractor can prevent many medical issues from developing and will keep your spine strong and your body healthy.

Dr. Yvonne Rose Fedewa D.C. Website: www.elifeboise.com Health blog: www.essentiallifeboise.blogspot.com

Naturopathic Physician

Naturopathic medicine is a distinct system of primary health care, a practice of preventing, diagnosing, and treating conditions of the human mind and body.

Naturopathic physicians work with their patients to prevent and treat acute and chronic illness and disease, restore health, and establish optimal fitness by supporting the person's inherent self-healing process. This is accomplished through...

- **Prevention.** Prevention of disease is emphasized through public health measures and hygiene as well as the encouragement and guidance to help clients adopt lifestyles that will help maintain optimal health.

- **Diagnosis.** Diagnosis and evaluation of the individual's state of health are accomplished by integrating traditional, clinical, and laboratory diagnostic methods.

- **Treatment and care.** Therapeutic methods and substances are used that work in harmony with the person's inherent self-help process, including dietetics and nutritional substances; botanical medicine; psychotherapy; naturopathic physical medicine, manipulative therapy, and obstetrics (natural childbirth); minor surgery; prescription medications; homeopathy; and acupuncture. For more information, go to http://naturopathic.org/

Lessons I've Learned in My Life!

I used to think the worst thing in life was to end up all alone. It's not. The worst thing in life is to end up with people who make you feel all alone. Pick your friends wisely.

Homeopathic Physician What Is Homeopathy?

Homeopathy, also known as homeopathic medicine, is a whole medical system that originated in Europe and has been practiced in the United States since the early nineteenth century. Homeopathy is based on three principles:

- **Like cures like.** Homeopathy demonstrates that a substance that produces a certain set of symptoms in a healthy person can cure a sick person experiencing those same symptoms. For instance, onions make your eyes water when you cut them. If you have a cold or allergies and your symptoms include a runny nose, the likely remedy to treat your runny nose would be Allium Cepa, which is made from onions.

- **Minimum dose.** Unlike conventional medicines, a homeopathic medicine is believed to be more effective when its active ingredient is diluted and succussed (shaken vigorously). Data indicates that the homeopathic medicine gains increased effectiveness with each additional dilution-succession step. Furthermore, the safety profile of the medicine increases with increased dilution.

- **Individualized medicines.** Ideally, homeopathic treatment is tailored to each person. In this case, practitioners select medicines according to a total picture of the patient, including physical symptoms but also lifestyle, emotional and mental states, and other factors.

Why Homeopathy?

Developed by pharmacists, homeopathic medicines are strong in relieving symptoms but gentle in the way they work. They are 100 percent natural with no drug interactions and non-habit-forming. They can be taken by nearly anyone at any time, from infants to the elderly, including anyone taking prescription medications. They have a high margin of safety. They can be given to young children without fear of misdosing or overdosing.

Chapter 11 Review

1. How would a patient benefit by seeing either a functional or environmental doctor?

_____

_____

_____

2. Why is chiropractic important to your health care?

_____

_____

_____

3. What are the benefits of a naturopathic physician?

_____

_____

_____

4. What are the benefits of a homeopathic physician?

_____

_____

_____

12

MY DETOX DRAGON

S ometimes there aren't any trumpets, just lots of dragons. Sometimes there aren't any medals to win, no golden chalice. There's no honor in having fought a fierce dragon. Sometimes, all you can say is, "The day is gone, and I tried my best." Sometimes, the very best you can do is to keep trying. But whatever you do, don't give up.

Tomorrow is another day.

This isn't the end of my story, but it is the end of my book and the beginning of a new chapter to my life after a very long journey. This was a trip I didn't ask to take, and I wish I had a do-over, but sometimes we are given opportunities disguised as challenges. I wasn't totally alone. My husband Ron walked beside me every step of the way. He took me to my many doctor appointments and traveled with me to out-of-state doctors and hospitals for tests. He came to get me when I couldn't get home because my brain and legs decided not to work right. The year that I was president of Soroptimist, Ron had perfect attendance because he was at every meeting and event as my backup plan in case I had a problem and he needed to get me out of a meeting quickly. There was also my dear friend Darrel and his wife Dorothy, who were always so close, and I could count on them at the drop of a hat. The secret is now out after twenty-three years. How do I feel? Relief! Like a heavy load has been lifted from my shoulders. I have known that I have had a problem with toxic chemicals since 1990, but I couldn't find a doctor in the state I live in that would listen objectively. When I removed the toxic household products from my home in 2011, I started noticing subtle health improvements. Suddenly I made the connection that the problem wasn't just my initial contact with toxins but also my constant low-level exposure that was keeping me sick.

That knowledge inspired me to finally take a huge step, come out of the closet, and share my story. It didn't even cross my mind that someone else might have the same struggles that I had been going through. While researching the book, I actually discovered the final pieces of my puzzle. The neurological problem that would last three or four hours was neurotoxicity.

Then while finishing the last part of the book, I ran across a doctor in Atlanta who also wrote a book about toxins and has a protocol for removing toxins from the body. I made an appointment, flew to Atlanta, and had a very enlightening meeting with Dr. Kolb.

The testing showed mold in my brain. Since then, I found out my chiropractor had mold in her brain while she was in college. She said it took a very long time for her to remove the mold through a detox program and to regain her health.

So now as the book ends, my detox program begins to finally get rid of the problem that has held me back from doing activities with my grandkids, friends, and husband because of fear of the unknown.

I talked to a very nice man last night who bought something from me on Craigslist. We started talking about toxins because of the book. He said his wife had been having serious problems for years and had been to many doctors. But they couldn't seem to find anything wrong, and she was so frustrated. Can anyone relate to this story?

I said she was probably going to the wrong type of doctor, and I told him my story plus shared some information from *Your Toxic Enemy*. I'm going to give her a call.

Maybe—just maybe—I was given this challenge for a reason. Maybe I can help someone else along the way as he or she fights his or her fierce dragon and I might just make new friends.

Remember the saying, "Today is the first day of the rest of your life." While it makes a great slogan for T-shirts and buttons, there is also a lot of truth to it.

Albert Camus said, "Life is a sum total of all your choices." Remember that you're only one choice away from changing your life for the better. Join me in my quest for a healthier lifestyle. I promise to never take good health for granted again.

Lessons I've Learned in My Life!

Being kind is more important than being right. People will forget what you said and did, but people will never forget how you made them feel. Sometimes when you are angry, you have the right to be angry, but that doesn't give you the right to be cruel. Resolving conflict is better than avoiding it. That's when you harbor bitterness, and happiness will dock elsewhere. It's not always wise to say the first thing that pops into your head.

- http://leslietorburn.wordpress.com
- www.biomat4healing.biomat.com
- www.lifetimevibe.com/braintrainer
- www.plastikos.com
- www.lisanagy.con
- www.touchstoneessentials.com
- http://EzineArticles.com/?expert=Larry J White
- www.janethull.com
- www.melaleuca.com/judiedietzler
- http://hpd.nlm.nih.gov/index.htm
- www.healthy-communications.com/

- www.dfsgardenclub.org
- http://antiagingchoices.com/
- http://green.wikia.com/wiki/
  Toxins in Household Cleaning Products
- www.lacsd.org
- www.academyofwellness.com
- http://www.jingorb.com?ref=1120
- www.melauca.com/
- www.judiedietzler.com

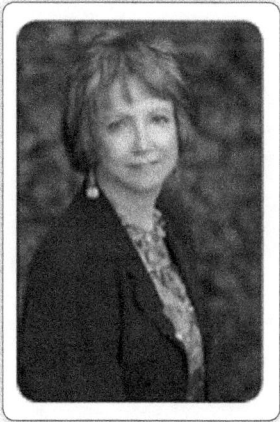

Judie Dietzler is an entrepreneur, trainer, public speaker, and Certified Hypnotherapist and Health Coach. Twenty-three years ago, she was exposed to a toxic chemical, losing her career and nearly her life in the process. This experience has led her to strive to provide clients with the tools needed to toxin-proof their environment and improve the quality of their life. This is her story, but it could be yours.

Author Photo by Cy Gilbert Photography

www.ingramcontent.com/pod-product-compliance
Lightning Source LLC
Chambersburg PA
CBHW031153020426
42333CB00013B/648